T0358854

New Postpartum Visit: Beginning of Lifelong Health

Editor

HAYWOOD L. BROWN

OBSTETRICS AND GYNECOLOGY CLINICS OF NORTH AMERICA

www.obgyn.theclinics.com

Consulting Editor
WILLIAM F. RAYBURN

September 2020 • Volume 47 • Number 3

ELSEVIER

1600 John F. Kennedy Boulevard • Suite 1800 • Philadelphia, Pennsylvania, 19103-2899

http://www.theclinics.com

OBSTETRICS AND GYNECOLOGY CLINICS OF NORTH AMERICA Volume 47, Number 3
September 2020 ISSN 0889-8545, ISBN-13: 978-0-323-79494-7

Editor: Kerry Holland
Developmental Editor: Kristen Helm

Obstetrics and Gynecology Clinics (ISSN 0889-8545) is published quarterly by Elsevier Inc., 360 Park Avenue South, New York, NY 10010-1710. Months of issue are March, June, September, and December. Periodicals postage paid at New York, NY, and additional mailing offices. Subscription price per year is $325.00 (US individuals), $719.00 (US institutions), $100.00 (US students), $404.00 (Canadian individuals), $908.00 (Canadian institutions), $100.00 (Canadian students), $459.00 (international individuals), $908.00 (international institutions), and $225.00 (international students). To receive student/resident rate, orders must be accompanied by name of affiliated institution, date of term, and the signature of program/residency coordinator on institution letterhead. Orders will be billed at individual rate until proof of status is received. Foreign air speed delivery is included in all *Clinics* subscription prices. All prices are subject to change without notice. POSTMASTER: Send address changes to *Obstetrics and Gynecology Clinics*, Elsevier Health Sciences Division, Subscription Customer Service, 3251 Riverport Lane, Maryland Heights, MO 63043. **Customer Service: Telephone: 1-800-654-2452 (U.S. and Canada); 314-447-8871 (outside U.S. and Canada). Fax: 314-447-8029. E-mail: journalscustomerservice-usa@elsevier.com (for print support); journalsonlinesupport-usa@elsevier. com (for online support).**

Reprints. For copies of 100 or more of articles in this publication, please contact the Commercial Reprints Department, Elsevier Inc., 360 Park Avenue South, New York, New York 10010-1710. Tel.: 212-633-3874; Fax: 212-633-3820; E-mail: reprints@elsevier.com.

Obstetrics and Gynecology Clinics of North America is also published in Spanish by McGraw-Hill Interamericana Editores S.A., P.O. Box 5-237, 06500, Mexico; in Portuguese by Reichmann and Affonso Editores, Rio de Janeiro, Brazil; and in Greek by Paschalidis Medical Publications, Athens, Greece.

Obstetrics and Gynecology Clinics of North America is covered in *MEDLINE/PubMed (Index Medicus), Excerpta Medica, Current Concepts/Clinical Medicine, Science Citation Index, BIOSIS, CINAHL, and ISI/BIOMED.*

Contributors

CONSULTING EDITOR

WILLIAM F. RAYBURN, MD, MBA
Associate Dean, Continuing Medical Education and Professional Development, Distinguished Professor and Emeritus Chair, Obstetrics and Gynecology, University of New Mexico School of Medicine, Albuquerque, New Mexico, USA

EDITOR

HAYWOOD L. BROWN, MD
Professor of Obstetrics and Gynecology, Associate Dean, Diversity, Morsani College of Medicine, Vice President Institutional Equity, University of South Florida, Tampa, Florida, USA

AUTHORS

HAYWOOD L. BROWN, MD
Professor of Obstetrics and Gynecology, Associate Dean, Diversity, Morsani College of Medicine, Vice President Institutional Equity, University of South Florida, Tampa, Florida, USA

AARON B. CAUGHEY, MD, PhD
Department Chair of Obstetrics and Gynecology, Oregon Health & Science University, Portland, Oregon, USA

NATHANIEL DeNICOLA, MD, MSHP
Department of Obstetrics and Gynecology, The George Washington University, Washington, DC, USA

SERINA FLOYD, MD, MSPH
Medical Director, Planned Parenthood of Metropolitan Washington, DC, Washington, DC, USA; Assistant Professor, Office of Educational Affairs, University of Virginia School of Medicine, Charlottesville, Virginia, USA

KABONI W. GONDWE, PhD, GH, UCM, RN
Assistant Professor, UW Milwaukee College of Nursing, External Member, Center for Advancing Population Science, Medical College of Wisconsin, Milwaukee, Wisconsin, USA

EMILY B. KROSKA, PhD
Clinical Assistant Professor, Department of Psychological and Brain Sciences, University of Iowa, Iowa City, Iowa, USA

JAMIE O. LO, MD
Assistant Professor, Department of Obstetrics and Gynecology, Oregon Health & Science University, Portland, Oregon, USA

JUDETTE M. LOUIS, MD, MPH
James Ingram Professor and Chair, Department of Obstetrics and Gynecology, University of South Florida, Tampa, Florida, USA

ADETOLA F. LOUIS-JACQUES, MD
Assistant Professor, Division of Maternal Fetal Medicine, Department of Obstetrics and Gynecology, Morsani College of Medicine, University of South Florida Tampa, Florida, USA

ANA REBECCA MEEKINS, MD
Fellow in Female Pelvic Medicine and Reconstructive Surgery, Department of Obstetrics and Gynecology, Division of Urogynecology, Duke University School of Medicine, Durham, North Carolina, USA

JESSICA M. PAGE, MD
Visiting Instructor, Fellow in Maternal-Fetal Medicine, Department of Obstetrics and Gynecology, University of Utah Health, Salt Lake City, Utah, USA

PEERAYA SAWANGKUM, MD
Department of Obstetrics and Gynecology, University of South Florida, Tampa, Florida, USA

NAZEMA Y. SIDDIQUI, MD, MHS
Associate Professor, Department of Obstetrics and Gynecology, Division of Urogynecology, Duke University School of Medicine, Durham, North Carolina, USA

ROBERT M. SILVER, MD
John A. Dixon Endowed Presidential Professor and Chair, Department of Obstetrics and Gynecology, University of Utah Health, Salt Lake City, Utah, USA

MARIA J. SMALL, MD, MPH
Associate Professor, Department of Obstetrics and Gynecology, Duke University, Division of Maternal Fetal Medicine, Duke University School of Medicine, Duke University Medical Center, Durham, North Carolina, USA

GRAEME N. SMITH, MD, PhD
Professor and Head, Department of Obstetrics and Gynecology, Queen's University, Kingston, Ontario, Canada

ZACHARY N. STOWE, MD
Professor, Department of Psychiatry, University of Wisconsin-Madison, Madison, Wisconsin, USA

ALISON M. STUEBE, MD, MSc
Professor, Division of Maternal Fetal Medicine, Department of Obstetrics and Gynecology, The University of North Carolina at Chapel Hill, Department of Maternal and Child Health, Carolina Global Breastfeeding Institute, Gillings School of Global Public Health, Chapel Hill, North Carolina, USA

SYDNEY M. THAYER, MD
Obstetrics and Gynecology Resident Physician, Department of Obstetrics and Gynecology, Oregon Health & Science University, Portland, Oregon, USA

MARGARET S. VILLERS, MD, MSCR
Maternal-Fetal Medicine, Mary Washington Medical Group, Fredericksburg, Virginia, USA

Contents

healthy weight between pregnancies by improving gestational weight gain. These interventions include lifestyle behavioral changes, diet and exercise, and motivational interviewing.

Perinatal care, including the management of mental health issues, often falls under the auspices of primary care providers. Postpartum depression (PPD) is a common problem that affects up to 15% of women. Most women at risk can be identified before delivery based on psychiatric history, symptoms during pregnancy, and recent psychosocial stressors. Fortunately, there have been a variety of treatment studies using antidepressants, nonpharmacologic interactions, and most recently, allopregnanolone (Brexanolone) infusion that have shown benefits. The most commonly used screening scale, Edinburgh Postnatal Depression Scale, a 10-item self-rated scale, has been translated into a variety of languages.

Pregnant and postpartum women with opiate use disorder present a challenge in perinatal care. It is important for health care teams to provide sensitive and compassionate evidence-based care for these women, who often are stigmatized during the prenatal, delivery, and postpartum periods. Women with opiate use disorder are at risk for inadequate prenatal and postpartum care and for complications. Infants are at risk for neonatal abstinence syndrome and are expected to require neonatal intensive care. Pain management during labor and for cesarean delivery requires consultation and collaboration with providers who have expertise in management of addiction. Postpartum follow-up is essential.

Cesarean delivery (CD) wound complications disrupt the time a mother spends with her newborn. Surgical site infections (SSI) may result in unplanned office visits, emergency room visits, and hospital readmissions. Despite increasing attention to preoperative preparation, the CD SSI rate remains high. Local practices must be evaluated, and new methods to reduce CD SSI must be used.

A systematic, effective stillbirth evaluation is important for identification of potential causes of fetal death. Knowledge of potential causes of fetal death facilitates emotional closure for patients and informs recurrence risk as well as future pregnancy management. The highest-yield components of a stillbirth evaluation for finding a cause of fetal death are fetal autopsy, placental pathology, and genetic testing. All patients should be offered these tests following a stillbirth. A clear plan for postpartum follow-up should be made with the patient in order to ensure ongoing support through the grief and recovery process.

Maria J. Small, Kaboni W. Gondwe, and Haywood L. Brown

Post-traumatic stress disorder (PTSD) accompanies miscarriage, intrauterine fetal demise, and preterm birth. Levels of PTSD may be higher for women who experience acute, life-threatening events during labor and delivery. Severe maternal morbidities or near misses for maternal death disproportionately impact African American, Hispanic, American Indian, and women in rural communities. Expanding research demonstrates association between severe maternal morbidity or near-miss events and PTSD. Multiple preceding conditions and intrapartum and postpartum events place women at higher risk for PTSD. Postpartum evaluation provides an opportunity for PTSD screening. Untreated perinatal PTSD impacts long-term maternal and child health and contributes to health disparities.

Serina Floyd

Pregnancy and the postpartum period are ideal times for health care providers to identify and address the contraceptive needs and desires of patients. In addition to the opportunity to promote healthy pregnancy spacing, individuals can also be cared for at a time when it is convenient, they have access to health care, and they are motivated to prevent repeat pregnancy. Patient-centered care using a shared medical decision-making framework can not only promote positive patient-provider interactions but also increase positive outcomes. Comprehensive provision of information on all methods and identification of contraceptive preferences can help patients select the best option.

Ana Rebecca Meekins and Nazema Y. Siddiqui

Pelvic floor disorders are common in the postpartum period. These disorders can significantly affect one's quality of life during a period that is already filled with emotional and physiologic change. This review focuses on the presentation, diagnosis, and treatment of the 3 major pelvic floor disorders in postpartum women, namely, urinary incontinence, fecal incontinence, and pelvic organ prolapse.

Haywood L. Brown and Graeme N. Smith

Heart disease is the leading cause of mortality in adult women. Beyond the traditional risk factors of obesity, diabetes, and hypercholesterolemia, women with the pregnancy complications of preeclampsia, gestational diabetes, prematurity, and low birth weight for gestational age (fetal growth restriction) are at higher risk for later development of cardiovascular disease. Education of women and providers about the association of

OBSTETRICS AND GYNECOLOGY CLINICS

SERIES OF RELATED INTEREST

Clinics in Perinatology
www.perinatology.theclinics.com
Pediatric Clinics of North America
www.pediatrics.theclinics.com

THE CLINICS ARE AVAILABLE ONLINE!
Access your subscription at:
www.theclinics.com

Foreword

The Postpartum Visit: An Optimal Time for Reflection and Looking Ahead

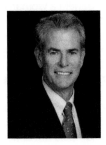

William F. Rayburn, MD, MBA
Consulting Editor

This issue of *Obstetrics and Gynecology Clinics of North America* pertains to the essential need of obstetricians and their coproviders to reexamine their practices for their postpartum patients. The issue is capably edited by Haywood L. Brown, MD, a past president of the American College of Obstetricians and Gynecologists, who had this as a principal focus during his recent presidency. We have accepted the puerperium as the time following delivery during which pregnancy-induced maternal anatomic and physiologic changes return to the nonpregnant state. Standard texts describe well the involution of the reproductive tract, urinary tract, perineum and abdominal wall, blood and blood volume, and lactation and breastfeeding.

This issue goes beyond these standard descriptions, which are frequently in the first few days or month. The key element during this transition period is a comprehensive visit within the first 12 weeks. This visit is an optimal time to perform several essential tasks: review maternal and fetal adaptations to the recent pregnancy; perform a physical examination especially of any cesarean delivery surgical site and perineum; determine any needed screening or testing; counsel the patient on recommended lifestyle changes and health care interventions; and explain the transition back to well-woman care for surveillance and management of any adjustment difficulties.

At the postpartum visit, the obstetrician or other care provider should identify interval care recommendations for general and reproductive health promotion. This counseling includes a review of the patient's plan for the planning, spacing, and timing of the next pregnancy; discussion of vaccinations (eg, rubella, varicella, Tdap), and nutrition counseling and supplementation. Discussion should include inquiring and counseling about hazardous behaviors, such as sexually transmitted infections, tobacco, alcohol, and opiate or other substance use disorders.

Obstet Gynecol Clin N Am 47 (2020) xi–xii
https://doi.org/10.1016/j.ogc.2020.06.001
0889-8545/20/© 2020 Published by Elsevier Inc.

obgyn.theclinics.com

Although the puerperium is less complex than pregnancy, the puerperium represents appreciable changes, with some being either bothersome or worrisome to the new mother. Interconception care offers a valuable opportunity to improve a woman's health and any children she may have in the future. Although many contraceptive methods can be initiated immediately after delivery, the postpartum visit is an opportune time to discuss contraception options, especially long-acting reversible contraceptive methods.

Many new mothers face challenges beyond the first 2 months that may require social support, lactation consultation, individualized education about newborn care, and emotional support. Screening for depression has the potential to benefit a woman and her family. If this persists or develops into clinically significant depression, anxiety, or posttraumatic stress, intervention would be necessary. Women with limited resources or inadequate insurance, who are enrolled in Medicaid, who are living in rural communities, or who are undocumented immigrants encounter difficulties that prohibit accessing care. The final article in this issue, pertaining to the role of telemedicine in postpartum follow-up, is especially helpful.

This issue reexamines the persistence or recurrence of many medical and obstetric conditions during pregnancy. Morbid obesity, gestational diabetes, hypertension, and heart disease are highlighted. As an example, women with preeclampsia are almost 4 times more likely to develop diabetes and almost 12 times more likely to develop hypertension that requires medication. Up to 70% of women with gestational diabetes develop type 2 diabetes mellitus within 5 years. Depending on the pregnancy outcome, it would be worthwhile to discuss recurrence risks and implications of any fetal growth restriction, preterm birth, fetal anomalies, stillbirth, and other conditions well before any future pregnancy. I concur with Dr Brown's recommendation for a follow-up annual evaluation for those who those at risk of a recurrent pregnancy complication or near-miss morbidity.

I appreciate the efforts of Dr Brown and his team of experienced obstetricians for their timely, thoughtful, and comprehensive recommendations about the many topics mentioned above. Regardless of whether the patient's subsequent well-woman care is provided by the same caregiver who attended her delivery, an internist, a family physician, or another health care provider, it is important to clearly identify any needed follow-up care or referrals. An accurate communication of timely information during a patient handoff from 1 member of the health care team to another is critical for more optimal care and safety.

William F. Rayburn, MD, MBA
Department of Obstetrics and Gynecology
University of New Mexico School of Medicine
MSC 10 5580, 1 University of New Mexico
Albuquerque, NM 87131-0001, USA

E-mail address:
wrayburnmd@gmail.com

Preface

Changing the Postpartum Care Paradigm

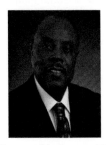

Haywood L. Brown, MD
Editor

Postpartum follow-up for all women after childbirth is essential for the mother, for the baby, and for long-term health. While the initial postpartum visit should address recovery from childbirth, lactation, and contraception concerns, it should be recognized as an opportunity to evaluate for mental health, labor outcome and complications, perineal rehabilitation, and ultimately, long-term health. Approximately 60% of all maternal deaths occur postpartum, and early follow-up is important for those most vulnerable, such as women at risk for thromboembolic and cardiovascular morbidity and mortality. Lack of postpartum follow-up contributes to disparities in maternal and infant mortality and early breast-feeding discontinuation and is a missed opportunity for education on recurrence risk for pregnancy complications, such as preeclampsia, prematurity, gestational diabetes, and adverse perinatal outcomes. It is also a missed opportunity for nutrition, exercise, and contraception counseling, which are essential for interconception and overall well women's health. Women with limited resources, those on Medicaid, and those from rural communities who have challenges with access are less likely to seek postpartum care.

This emphasis on the postpartum follow-up visit should include a contact assessment within the first 3 weeks after delivery followed by a comprehensive visit within 12 weeks postpartum, which provides an opportunity for mental health assessment and reproductive life planning. In addition, follow-up is recommended at 12 months for ongoing care, particularly for those women at risk of medical conditions and for those who have experienced a pregnancy complication or a near-miss pregnancy-related morbidity that impacts long-term health.

Obstet Gynecol Clin N Am 47 (2020) xiii–xiv
https://doi.org/10.1016/j.ogc.2020.06.002
0889-8545/20/© 2020 Published by Elsevier Inc.

obgyn.theclinics.com

In order to achieve this goal of a more comprehensive postpartum care model, insurance coverage must be extended beyond the traditional 6-week period, and education on postpartum guidelines should be disseminated to patients, providers, and payers.

Haywood L. Brown, MD
Diversity, Inclusion & Equal Opportunity
University of South Florida
13101 Bruce B. Downs Blvd
MDC 3rd floor
Tampa, FL 33612, USA

E-mail address:
haywoodb@usf.edu

Enabling Breastfeeding to Support Lifelong Health for Mother and Child

Adetola F. Louis-Jacques, MD[a],*, Alison M. Stuebe, MD, MSc[b,c]

KEYWORDS

- Lactation • Breastfeeding • Breastfeeding benefits • Breastfeeding disparities
- Breastfeeding recommendations • Lactation challenges

KEY POINTS

- Breastfeeding is associated with improved health outcomes for mothers and children.
- Given the significant health impact of breastfeeding, national organizations recommend exclusive breastfeeding for 6 months and continued breastfeeding for at least 1 year, in combination with complementary foods.
- Breastfeeding rates are increasing in the United States; however, structural factors cause significant disparities by sociodemographic status. Non-Hispanic black mothers have the lowest breastfeeding rates of any racial/ethnic group.
- These breastfeeding inequities may contribute to other inequities in maternal child health outcomes.
- Many women experience challenges with breastfeeding, and obstetrician-gynecologists are well positioned to protect, promote, and support breastfeeding.

INTRODUCTION
Benefits

Breastfeeding is associated with improved health outcomes for mothers and children.[1–5] Short-term benefits for mothers include a decreased risk of postpartum hemorrhage[6] and prolonged amenorrhea in mothers who exclusively or predominantly breastfeed in the first 6 months postpartum.[7] The relationship between breastfeeding and postpartum depression seems to be bidirectional: among women without a prenatal diagnosis of depression, high positive emotions during infant feeding were

[a] Division of Maternal Fetal Medicine, Department of Obstetrics and Gynecology, University of South Florida Morsani College of Medicine, 2 Tampa General Circle, 6th Floor, Tampa, FL 33606, USA; [b] Division of Maternal Fetal Medicine, Department of Obstetrics and Gynecology, University of North Carolina, Chapel Hill, NC, USA; [c] Department of Maternal and Child Health, Carolina Global Breastfeeding Institute, Gillings School of Global Public Health, 3010 Old Clinic Building, CB #7516, Chapel Hill, NC 27599, USA
* Corresponding author.
E-mail address: alouisjacques@usf.edu

Obstet Gynecol Clin N Am 47 (2020) 363–381
https://doi.org/10.1016/j.ogc.2020.04.001
0889-8545/20/© 2020 Elsevier Inc. All rights reserved.

obgyn.theclinics.com

associated with lower depression symptoms at 2, 6, and 12 months.[8] However, mothers who face breastfeeding challenges or do not meet their breastfeeding goals have increased risk of developing postpartum depression.[2]

In terms of long-term health outcomes, breastfeeding is associated with decreased maternal risk of metabolic syndrome, type 2 diabetes mellitus, and cardiovascular disease, in particular, hypertension.[1–3,5,9–11] Breast, ovarian, endometrial, and thyroid cancers have also been reported to be lower in breastfeeding mothers.[11–13] Some of these benefits are dose dependent (exclusive vs partial vs none), and in general, the longer a woman lactates during her reproductive years the greater the association with improved lifelong health.

For children, breastfeeding is associated with a decreased risk of otitis media, gastroenteritis, respiratory tract infections, inflammatory bowel disease, obesity, diabetes mellitus, asthma, childhood leukemia, and sudden infant death syndrome.[1–3,14] Preterm infants who receive an exclusive human milk diet have a lower risk of developing necrotizing enterocolitis,[1] and preterm infants who receive human milk have higher neurodevelopment scores as toddlers.[15]

On a population level, enabling breastfeeding has considerable impact. In a simulation model comparing current breastfeeding rates with optimal breastfeeding rates, described as 90% of mothers exclusively breastfeeding each child for 6 months and continuing through 12 months, current, suboptimal breastfeeding practices incurred an excess of 2619 premature maternal deaths (95% confidence interval [CI] 1978–3259) and 721 child deaths (95% CI 543–899) and $3 billion in medical costs and $1.2 billion in nonmedical costs.[3] In addition, feeding breast milk substitutes has environmental costs: an analysis of the carbon footprint of breast milk substitute production and preparation[16] found that 6 months of breastfeeding saves between 95 and 153 kg of CO_2 compared with formula feeding.[17]

However, there are important methodological issues to consider. Randomizing women to breastfeed or formula feed is unethical, thus, most studies are observational. There are sociodemographic differences between mothers who breastfeed and those who do not breastfeed: breastfeeding mothers are more likely to be white, older, leaner, married, and have higher income levels.[4] Furthermore, poor maternal baseline metabolic health such as obesity, gestational diabetes may decrease attained breastfeeding duration and exclusivity.[18] Lastly, breastfeeding definitions vary between studies. However, the preponderance of the evidence demonstrates that enabling women to breastfeed improves outcomes for mothers, children, and the planet.

CONTENT
Recommendations and Contraindications

Given the health impact of breastfeeding, health organizations recommend exclusive breastfeeding for 6 months and continued breastfeeding for at least 1 year, or longer as mutually desired, in combination with complementary foods.[1,14,19] Most mothers are able to breastfeed their infants; however, there are a few contraindications to breastfeeding and or providing their expressed milk to infants[20] (refer to **Table 1**).

When mothers need to temporarily discontinue breastfeeding, health care providers should arrange follow-up consultation or instructions on when they are able to resume breastfeeding. The mothers should also receive lactation support on how to express and discard their milk in order to maintain their supply. For those with airborne and contact precautions, temporary separation of the mother and infant may be required; however, expressed breast milk can be given to the infant by another provider.

Table 1
Contraindications to breastfeeding and/or feeding of breast milk

Mothers should NOT breastfeed or feed expressed breast milk to their infants	• Classic galactosemia in the infant • Mothers actively using illicit street drug, such as PCP or cocaine • Mothers infected with HIV[a], human T-cell lymphotropic virus type I or type II • Mothers with confirmed or suspected Ebola virus disease

Mothers should temporarily NOT breastfeed or feed expressed breast milk to their infants	• Mother is infected with untreated brucellosis
	• Mother is taking certain medications, for example, certain chemotherapies
	• The mother is undergoing diagnostic imaging with radiopharmaceuticals
	• Mother has an active herpes simplex virus infection with lesions present on the breast (transmission)
	  ○ She may feed or provide expressed milk from the unaffected breast provided the lesions on the affected breast are covered.
	  ○ She may resume feeding or providing expressed milk from the affected breast once the lesions have resolved.

Mothers should temporarily NOT breastfeed, but CAN feed expressed breast milk	• Mother has untreated, active tuberculosis ○ She may resume breastfeeding after 2 wk of appropriate treatment and she is no longer contagious • Active varicella that developed within 5 d prior or 2 d after delivery

Abbreviations: HIV, human immunodeficiency virus; PCP, phencyclidine.
[a] HIV recommendation only applies to the United States.
Adapted from Centers for Disease Control and Prevention (CDC). Contraindications to Breastfeeding or Feeding Expressed Breast Milk to Infants. Available at: https://www.cdc.gov/breastfeeding/breastfeeding-special-circumstances/contraindications-to-breastfeeding.html. Accessed Dec 14 2019.

National Breastfeeding Rates and Sociodemographic Disparities

Breastfeeding rates are increasing in the United States,[21] (**Fig. 1**), and 5 of the 8 2020 Healthy People Goals established by the US Department of Health and Human Services[22] have been achieved (**Table 2**). However, there are significant disparities by sociodemographic status. Asian American mothers have the highest breastfeeding rates, and they, along with Non-Hispanic White mothers, have successfully surpassed the 2020 Healthy People goals.[23] Although Hispanic mothers have exceeded the initiation goals, they have not met the sustained or exclusive Healthy People goals.[23] There has been improvement in breastfeeding rates among Non-Hispanic Black women.[21,23] Despite these gains, Non-Hispanic black mothers have the lowest breastfeeding rates of any racial/ethnic group (**Table 3**),[23] and the disparity persists regardless of income or education status.[24]

In addition, low-income mothers who participate in the Special Supplemental Nutrition Program for Women, Infants, and Children (WIC) have lower breastfeeding rates when compared with mothers who are ineligible for WIC. Women who are older than or equal to 30 years, have a higher education, and are married are more likely to breastfeed. These sociodemographic disparities in infant feeding behaviors represent inequities and are a major public health concern. These breastfeeding inequities may

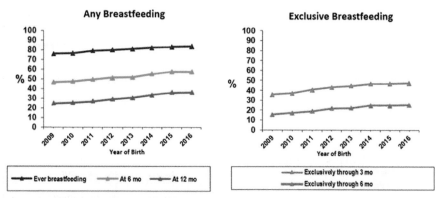

Fig. 1. Population impact of enabling optimal breastfeeding. Percentage of US children who were breastfed, by birth year. (*From* Centers for Disease Control and Prevention (CDC). Breastfeeding Rates. National Immunization Survey (NIS). Available at: https://www.cdc.gov/breastfeeding/data/nis_data/results.html. Accessed Dec 13 2019.)

Table 2			
Healthy people 2020 breastfeeding objectives			
	Healthy People 2020 Objectives	**Target (%)**	**Current Rates (%)[a]**
MICH[b]-21.1	Increase the proportion of infants who are breastfed: Ever	81.9	83.8 ✓
MICH-21.2	Increase the proportion of infants who are breastfed: At 6 mo	60.6	57.3
MICH-21.3	Increase the proportion of infants who are breastfed: At 1 y	34.1	36.2 ✓
MICH-21.4	Increase the proportion of infants who are breastfed: Exclusively through 3 mo	46.2	47.5 ✓
MICH-21.5	Increase the proportion of infants who are breastfed: Exclusively through 6 mo	25.5	25.4
MICH-22	Increase the proportion of employers who have worksite lactation support programs.	38.0	49.0 ✓
MICH-23	Reduce the proportion of breastfed newborns who receive formula supplementation within the first 2 d of life.	14.2	17.2
MICH-24	Increase the proportion of live births that occur in facilities that provide recommended care for lactating mothers and their babies.	8.1	26.1 ✓

[a] MICH-21 and MICH-23 current rates represent babies born in 2016 National Immunization Survey; MICH-22 current rates represent employers providing an on-site lactation/mother's room, Society for Human Resource Management, 2018 survey; MICH-24 current rates represent babies born in Baby-Friendly Hospitals and Birth Centers designated as of June 2018, Baby-Friendly USA.
[b] Maternal Infant and Child Health.
From Centers for Disease Control and Prevention (CDC). Breastfeeding Report Card: United States, 2018. Available at: https://www.cdc.gov/breastfeeding/data/reportcard.htm. Accessed Dec 13 2019.

Table 3
Rates of any and exclusive breastfeeding by race/ethnicity among children born in 2016

	Any Breastfeeding (BF) (%)			Exclusive Breastfeeding (EBF) (%)	
	Ever BF	BF at 6 mo	BF at 12 mo	EBF Through 3 mo	EBF Through 6 mo
Hispanic	82.9	51.6	32.1	42.0	20.4
Non-Hispanic White	86.6	61	39.6	52.9	29.1
Non-Hispanic Black	74.0	48.6	27.1	39.1	20.7
Non-Hispanic Asian	88.2	72.1	51.6	48.1	31.8

Adapted from Centers for Disease Control and Prevention (CDC). Rates of Any and Exclusive Breastfeeding by Socio-demographics among Children Born in 2016. Available at: https://www.cdc.gov/breastfeeding/data/nis_data/rates-any-exclusive-bf-socio-dem-2016.htm. Accessed Dec 14 2019.

contribute to other inequities in maternal child health outcomes throughout the life course.[25,26]

Role of the Obstetrician-Gynecologist

The health benefits of breastfeeding are well documented, and more than 80% of US women initiate breastfeeding; however, mothers in the United States face substantial challenges in meeting their personal breastfeeding goals, with approximately 60% weaning earlier than they had intended.[27] Reasons for premature weaning include but are not limited to perceptions of low milk supply, nipple pain, concerns about infant weight, breast engorgement, mastitis, maternal medication use, obesity, depressive symptoms, work constraints, and efforts associated with pumping.[27,28] Enabling women to meet their breastfeeding goals is a public health priority, and infant feeding should be addressed as a modifiable health behavior, rather than a lifestyle choice,[5] with attention to the structural and social barriers that can prevent women from meeting their intentions. The obstetrician-gynecologist (OBGYN) is well positioned to protect, promote, and support breastfeeding. OBGYNs can (1) provide breastfeeding education and practical skills from preconception to the postpartum period, (2) assess breastfeeding concerns and provide anticipatory guidance and support, and (3) address and manage lactation challenges in the postpartum.[5]

Although obstetricians can play a major role in providing breastfeeding education, a lack of breastfeeding knowledge and breastfeeding management skills is an impediment to this role.[29,30] Because of lack of breastfeeding education, many physicians are unable to address breastfeeding needs of their patients. Only 25% of women in the postpartum period thought that their breastfeeding concerns were addressed during prenatal care.[31] Thus it is essential to provide breastfeeding training to health care providers in order to increase their breastfeeding knowledge, hospital compliance with evidence-based measures, and patients' breastfeeding rates.[32,33]

Lactation Physiology

To fully support breastfeeding mothers, it is important that OBGYNs understand lactation physiology. During puberty, increasing estrogen and progesterone levels stimulate breast duct growth and alveolar development respectively. Breast secretory differentiation accelerates during pregnancy, and lactocytes develop the capacity to produce milk (lactogenesis I). The progesterone withdrawal in the immediate postpartum period initiates secretory activation (lactogenesis II). The transition from colostrum to mature milk begins at approximately 2 days postpartum. Nipple stimulation leads to release of prolactin from the anterior pituitary and oxytocin from the posterior pituitary. Prolactin stimulates milk synthesis, and oxytocin triggers milk secretion (**Fig. 2**).[34]

The key components of successful breastfeeding are letdown, latch, and moving milk[35]:

Letdown
- Oxytocin triggers contractions of myoepithelial cells surrounding alveoli, transferring milk through breast ducts to the nipple-areolar complex.
- Can be triggered by the sound, sight, or smell of the infant and inhibited by pain and stress.

Latch
- The infant takes most of the nipple and areola into his or her mouth, and little or no areola is visualized (**Fig. 3**).
- The infant's lips flange out.
- The latch is comfortable.

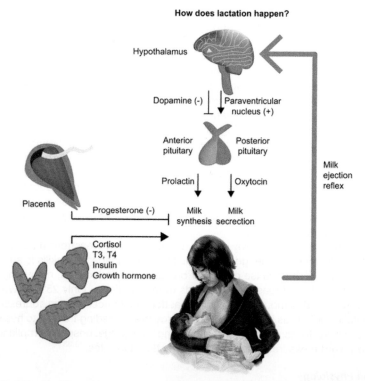

How does lactation happen?

Fig. 2. Physiology of lactation. During pregnancy, placental progesterone blocks milk synthesis. After birth, falling progesterone levels trigger onset of milk production. Infant suckling stimulates release of prolactin and oxytocin, which regulate milk synthesis and milk secretion. Cortisol, thyroid hormone, insulin, and growth hormone further support milk synthesis. (*From* Stuebe AM. Enabling women to achieve their breastfeeding goals. Obstet Gynecol 2014;123(3):644; with permission.)

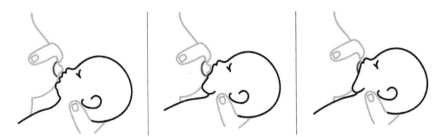

Fig. 3. Illustration of a good latch. (*From* Office on Women's Health (OWH). Learning to breastfeed. Getting a good latch. Available at: https://www.womenshealth.gov/breastfeeding/learning-breastfeed/getting-good-latch. Accessed Dec 13 2019.)

- The nipple is round after feeding. A compressed nipple indicates a poor latch and may lead to reduction in milk transfer and nipple trauma.

Moving milk

- Sustains milk production.
- To sustain lactation, mothers should drain their breasts 8 to 12 times per day via breastfeeding or express by hand or with a mechanical pump.

Preconception Counseling

Most women make their feeding choice before pregnancy or in the first trimester of pregnancy. The annual office encounter and other preconception visits are opportunities to discuss breastfeeding. The provider may obtain the patient's breastfeeding history and perform a breast examination to identify any structural or surgical problems. These visits provide an opportunity for counseling, anticipatory guidance, and to suggest modifications (eg, weight management, medication changes) that can help a mother successfully breastfeed.[36]

Prenatal Care

Counseling should begin early in the prenatal care with open-ended questions. Targeted education can subsequently be provided to address her concerns. See ACOG Physician Conversation Guide on Support for Breastfeeding for examples of questions and suggestions for education. Prenatal breastfeeding education by health care professionals can be augmented by lactation specialists, prenatal classes, breastfeeding support groups, and internet-based resources[5,36,37] (**Box 1**). Posters, videos, and pamphlets may also be used. The ACOG breastfeeding toolkit is an excellent resource for health care providers, with both patient and provider educational materials.[38]

When specific concerns regarding successful breastfeeding are raised, referral to a breastfeeding medicine specialist or to a lactation specialist may be beneficial to improve breastfeeding success. Examples include suspected cleft palate, previous negative breastfeeding experiences such as nipple trauma, or anatomic concerns such as prior breast reduction surgery or tubular breasts.

Intrapartum Care and the "Ten Steps to Successful Breastfeeding"

Intrapartum care

As a general rule, easier labor and birth are associated with easier initiation of breastfeeding. A longitudinal study of first-time mothers in California[39] quantified associations between intrapartum care and early feeding outcomes and identified several

---

Box 1
Breastfeeding resources for providers and patients

Providers

Educational Materials
- American College of Obstetricians and Gynecologists Breastfeeding Toolkit: http://www.acog.org/About-ACOG/ACOG-Departments/Toolkits-for-Health-Care-Providers/Breastfeeding-Toolkit
- *The CDC Guide to Strategies to Support Breastfeeding Mothers and Babies*: https://www.cdc.gov/breastfeeding/pdf/BF-Guide-508.PDF
- American Academy of Pediatrics Breastfeeding Education Resources: https://www.aap.org/en-us/advocacy-and-policy/aap-health-initiatives/Breastfeeding/Pages/Breastfeeding-Educational-Resources.aspx
- Well-Start International self-study modules: www.wellstart.org
- Schanler, Richard J., Krebs, Nancy and colleagues 2013. *Breastfeeding Handbook for Physicians, 2nd Edition*. Elk Grove Village, IL: American Academy of Pediatrics; Washington, DC: American College of Obstetricians and Gynecologists.
- Academy of Breastfeeding Medicine Protocols https://www.bfmed.org/protocols

Medication Use
- LactMed: https://www.ncbi.nlm.nih.gov/books/NBK501922/
- Organization of Teratology Information Specialists: https://mothertobaby.org/
- Infant Risk Center: https://www.infantrisk.com/

Mothers
- Office on Women's Health in the US Department of Health and Human Services: https://www.womenshealth.gov/breastfeeding

African American Mothers:
- US Department of Health and Human Services campaign to support breastfeeding for African American women: www.womenshealth.gov/itsonlynatural/
- Reaching Our Sisters Everywhere (ROSE): http://www.breastfeedingrose.org/
- Black Mothers Breastfeeding Association: http://blackmothersbreastfeeding.org

Blogs:
http://mochamanual.com
https://blackwomendobreastfeed.org

American Indian/Alaska Native mothers:
- Navajo Nation Breastfeeding Coalition: https://www.facebook.com/pg/Navajo-Nation-Breastfeeding-Coalition-275985218770/about/
- Native Breastfeeding Coalition of Washington: https://www.facebook.com/NABCWA/
- Native Mothering blog: http://nativemothering.com/

Hispanic/Latina mothers
- Lactancia Latina: http://www.breastfeedinghousecalls.com/lactancia-latinacom.html
- MHP Salud serving migrant mothers in Michigan, Texas, Florida, Ohio, and Washington: www.mhpsalud.org/programs/our-programs/instinto-maternal-program/

---

risk factors associated with suboptimal infant breastfeeding behavior on day 0 of life, including primiparity, cesarean birth, regional anesthesia, and a maternal interval greater than 18 hours without sleep. In a logistic regression analysis, flat or inverted nipples, primiparity, and cesarean birth were independent predictors of suboptimal infant breastfeeding behavior. For women birthing by c-section, targeted support[40] can improve outcomes. At birth, placing the infant skin-to-skin with the mother until the end of the first breastfeeding is a powerful intervention to enable breastfeeding. In the most recent Cochrane meta-analysis of randomized controlled trials, skin-to-skin care increased breastfeeding duration by 64 days (95% CI 37.8–89.5).[41]

During the maternity stay, keeping the mother and infant (rooming-in) together enables physiologic on-cue, frequent feeding.[42] It is helpful to talk about the rationale for rooming-in during antenatal care so that families are aware that infants are not typically cared for in a separate nursery at night. For women who have a medical need for sleep—such as those with a seizure disorder or psychiatric illness that is aggravated by sleep disruption—it can be helpful to ensure a support person is present to assist with nighttime care or make a plan for the infant to be cared for in the nursery for a period of time at night.

Ten steps to successful breastfeeding

The Ten Steps to successful breastfeeding contains a set of recommendations that protect, promote, and support breastfeeding in maternity and newborn care facilities. The "Ten Steps" were developed by the World Health Organization (WHO) and the United Nations Children's Fund in 1989, and they form the basis for the Baby Friendly Hospital Initiative. In 2017, WHO released updated guidelines[43](**Box 2**). Implementation of the Ten Steps increases the likelihood that women will initiate and sustain breastfeeding.[11] Maternity centers should implement this evidence-based care to enable mothers to meet their infant feeding goals.

Contraception

Interpregnancy intervals greater than 18 months are associated with improved outcomes for the subsequent pregnancy.[44] Obstetric providers should share this information with women to provide context for decisions about contraception following birth. Exclusive, frequent breastfeeding suppresses the hypothalamic-ovarian-pituitary axis and prevents pregnancy. Both the WHO[45] and the Centers for Disease

---

Box 2
Ten Steps to successful breastfeeding

Critical management procedures
1a. Comply fully with the *International Code of Marketing of Breast-milk Substitutes* and relevant World Health Assembly resolutions.
1b. Have a written infant feeding policy that is routinely communicated to staff and parents.
1c. Establish ongoing monitoring and data management systems.
2. Ensure that staff have sufficient knowledge, competence, and skills to support breastfeeding.

Key clinical practices
3. Discuss the importance and management of breastfeeding with pregnant women and their families.
4. Facilitate immediate and uninterrupted skin-to-skin contact and support mothers to initiate breastfeeding as soon as possible after birth.
5. Support mothers to initiate and maintain breastfeeding and manage common difficulties.
6. Do not provide breastfed newborns any food or fluids other than breast milk, unless medically indicated.
7. Enable mothers and their infants to remain together and to practice rooming-in 24 hours a day.
8. Support mothers to recognize and respond to their infants' cues for feeding.
9. Counsel mothers on the use and risks of feeding bottles, teats, and pacifiers.
10. Coordinate discharge so that parents and their infants have timely access to ongoing support and care.

From World Health Organization (WHO). Ten steps to successful breastfeeding. Available at: https://www.who.int/activities/promoting-baby-friendly-hospitals/ten-steps-to-successful-breastfeeding. Accessed April 5 2020; with permission.

Control and Prevention[46] Medical Eligibility Criteria for Contraception include the lactational amenorrhea method as an effective strategy for birth spacing. The risk of pregnancy is less than 2% for women who meet 3 criteria:

1. Amenorrhea;
2. Fully or nearly fully breastfeeding (no interval of >4–6 hours between breastfeeds); and
3. Less than 6 months postpartum.[47]

Obstetric providers should share these criteria with women so that they are aware of circumstances under which breastfeeding does, and does not, provide protection against pregnancy.

The impact of hormonal contraception on breastfeeding is controversial. Decreasing progesterone levels after delivery of the placenta coincide with onset of milk production,[48] and in theory, exogenous hormones could disrupt milk synthesis. Several studies have evaluated breastfeeding outcomes among women using progestin-only methods, and the extant data are reassuring[49]; however, these studies have been powered to detect fairly large effects, and most studies were limited to healthy mothers of term infants. As stated by American College of Obstetricians and Gynecologists, "Women considering immediate postpartum progestin-only contraception should be counseled about the theoretical risk of reduced duration of breastfeeding and about the preponderance of evidence that has not shown a negative effect on actual breastfeeding outcomes. Obstetric care providers should discuss any concerns within the context of each woman's desire to breastfeed and her risk of unplanned pregnancy, so that she can make an autonomous and informed decision.[5]" To support decision-making, obstetric care providers should ask open-ended questions about breastfeeding, birth spacing, and sexuality in order to support decision-making centered on the patient's values and preferences.[50]

Postpartum Care

The weeks following birth present multiple challenges for the new mother: she must recover from vaginal birth or cesarean, navigate shifting hormones, and learn to feed and care for the new infant.[51] Obstetric providers can assist women to navigate these challenges during antenatal care by helping women to craft a postpartum plan.[52] Planning starts with identifying family and friends who can provide material support in the weeks following birth. Anthropologists have shown that humans are collective breeders—we require the assistance of other adults, known as alloparents, to care for the new mother and infant. Although other primates have prehensile hands and feet that allow them to cling to their mothers' fur, human babies must be carried for at least the first year of life.[53] It really does "take a village" to nurture a human newborn. Obstetric care providers can encourage expectant mothers to identify support, including both given and chosen family, and explicitly plan for help with meals, care of siblings, and household tasks.

It can be helpful to explicitly discuss strategies for shared caregiving work in the context of exclusive breastfeeding. Although the mother is uniquely situated to feed the newborn, multiple caregivers can sooth, hold, swaddle, bathe, and diaper. For example, at night, some families find it helpful to "sleep in shifts": for a block of time, such as 6 PM to midnight, the mother is "off duty" except for feeding. When the infant cues to eat, another caregiver can gently wake the mother, assist with positioning the infant to nurse while side-lying, and, when the infant is finished, take the baby to burp, change, and settle while the mother goes back to sleep. This approach avoids engorgement from 6 hours without feeding, while enabling the mother to rest for a sustained period.

Some mothers elect to express milk so that other caregivers can bottle-feed the infant. It can be helpful to discuss the mother's goals to help inform when to start expressing and bottle feeding. Mechanical expression requires the mother's time, as well as time to prepare, wash and dry pump parts and bottles, and may not be less burdensome to the mother than direct breast feeding. Milk removal stimulates milk production, and frequent early mechanical expression may also lead to overproduction of milk, which can contribute to engorgement, plugged ducts, and mastitis. There is a paucity of evidence regarding strategies to begin expressing and storing milk in anticipation of the mother's return to work or school; expressing once a day, after the morning feed, is one commonly suggested approach.

Lactation Challenges

Many women experience challenges with breastfeeding, and as reproductive health providers, OBGYNs should be prepared to evaluate and manage breastfeeding difficulties. Such difficulties often co-present with postpartum depression; however, because of the stigma surrounding mental health, women may seek care for breastfeeding concerns and be reluctant to bring up anxiety or depression. Screening with a validated instrument, as well as asking open-ended questions, can be helpful to identify comorbid mood concerns.

Engorgement

Breast engorgement is the physiologic bilateral breast fullness that occurs most often between days 3 and 5 postpartum. This condition is typically a reassuring sign that secretion of mature milk has begun as part of lactogenesis II. The distention of the alveolar ducts with milk causes vascular and lymphatic compression. Factors associated with severely symptomatic breast engorgement may include primiparity, large amounts of intravenous fluids given in labor, history of premenstrual breast tenderness, and a history of breast surgery.[54] Women who had a cesarean delivery typically experience peak engorgement about 1 to 2 days later than women who had a vaginal birth.

Symptomatic engorgement may increase a woman's risk for early weaning and inadequate milk supply. There is insufficient evidence to recommend any specific treatment.[54,55] Severe engorgement may negatively affect the infant's ability to latch. Breast massage can be helpful[56]; additional treatment options include acupuncture, hot and cold packs, cabbage leaves, herbal remedies, minimal hand expression or pumping before feeds, acetaminophen, and ibuprofen.[55]

Nipple sensitivity and pain

Many women experience discomfort in the first 20 to 30 seconds of neonatal latch in the early postpartum period. Persistent discomfort or pain may lead to early weaning. Causes of persistent nipple pain are extensive and include latch problems, pump trauma, dermatoses, infection, vasospasm, allodynia or functional pain, oversupply or plugged ducts, and neonatal ankyloglossia.[57] A focused history and physical examination and evaluation of the latch may facilitate diagnosis. It is important to address the latch and other complications such as nipple trauma, superimposed infection, and vasospasm. Patients with persistent pain despite therapy should be referred to a lactation specialist.

Low milk supply

Mother's milk is sufficient for most infants. Yet, many women are concerned about their milk supply, and perceived low milk supply is one of the most common reasons for early weaning.[27,28] Feeding frequently (at least 8–12 times per day) will build milk supply. Mothers should be reassured if infants having frequent wet diapers are gaining weight steadily by day 5. If an actual low milk supply exists, she can often be supported to feed or express milk more frequently in order to increase her supply.[58]

Although most mothers can meet their infants' needs, some women cannot. Breastfeeding, as every other physiologic process, is not infallible.[59] Risk factors for lactation problems include primiparity, extremes of maternal age, obesity, history of breast reduction, and lack of noticeable breast enlargement during pregnancy.[60] Such risk factors should be communicated to the pediatric provider to ensure follow up within 24 to 48 hours of discharge. All families should be informed of signs and symptoms of dehydration such as worsening jaundice, inadequate wet or soiled diapers, lethargy, inconsolability, and infant stool that is not bright yellow by postpartum day 5.[58] Mothers with low milk supply may need to feed infants pasteurized donor milk or breastmilk substitutes when donor milk is not available.[58]

The most effective intervention to increase milk production is to increase milk removal, either by increasing the frequency of infant feeds or by mechanical milk expression. Galactagogues are drugs and herbs that are administered with the aim of improving milk supply.[61] Data to support efficacy for these agents are limited, at best. If women initiate galactagogues, it may be helpful to increase or decrease one herbal remedy at a time to allow assessment of which, if any, herbal preparation is helpful. Prescription medications proposed for increasing milk supply include dopamine antagonists, which increase prolactin levels, inhaled oxytocin, and metformin.[62] Domperidone is a prescription dopamine antagonist that modestly increases milk expression (meta-analysis 94 mL/d, 95% CI 71–117).[63] However, this drug is a QT interval prolonger and is not available in the United States due to concerns about adverse cardiac effects. Metoclopramide similarly is a dopamine antagonist, but side effects include depression, anxiety, and extrapyramidal effects[64]; close follow-up is therefore recommended if this drug is prescribed. Metformin is theorized to improve milk supply via increasing insulin sensitivity and has been tested in a single pilot randomized controlled trial that found a modest increase in milk production that was not statistically significant; 44% of the women randomized to metformin reported gastrointestinal side effects, and none wished to continue the study drug at the end of the trial.[65]

Given the paucity of therapeutic options for improving milk supply, some women who strongly desire to breastfeed may be unable to establish a full milk supply. OBGYNs and other obstetric providers should take time to explore a woman's feelings of frustration and disappointment and both validate her efforts and affirm that she is uniquely suited to decide what degree of effort is "worth it" to provide milk to her child. If mother and infant enjoy suckling at the breast, mothers can be advised that "You can nurture your baby at breast, no matter how much milk you make."

Mastitis

The clinical definition of mastitis includes fever, breast inflammation, and systemic signs. Risk factors include history of oversupply, nipple trauma, or prolonged milk stasis.[66] Dicloxacillin, 500 mg, four times a day for 10 to 14 days is the first-line outpatient therapy; for women allergic to penicillin, clindamycin, 300 mg, four times a day is recommended. The mother should be advised to continue breastfeeding or expressing milk during the treatment. Underlying risk factors should be addressed to prevent recurrent mastitis. Persistent infection should trigger an investigation for a breast abscess or methicillin-resistant *Staphylococcus aureus* infection. Abscess can be treated with ultrasound-guided drainage.

Preterm infants

Mother's milk serves as medication for preterm infants. It is important to share the importance of human milk and breastfeeding with mothers of preterm infants and to support them to initiate and sustain milk expression. Such counseling increases provision of breastfeeding without increasing maternal anxiety.[67] Mothers should be encouraged to initiate breastfeeding or expression of colostrum ideally within 6 hours of birth,[68] ideally within the first hour.[69] Patients should receive instructions on the benefits and mechanics of frequent hand expression with or without mechanical expression.[70] Preterm infants may have difficulty with learning how to effectively latch, suck, and swallow, so consultation with lactation specialists should be encouraged.

Medication use during lactation

Most medications are safe during lactation. Some mothers may choose not to initiate breastfeeding, wean earlier than intended, or not adhere with prescribed medications due to worries about medication use while breastfeeding.[71] Health care providers often incorrectly make recommendations regarding medication use during lactation.[72] Clinicians can base counseling on accurate and current data using resources such as the National Library of Medicine's LactMed database, Organization of Teratology Information Specialists (OTIS) Website www.mothertobaby.org, or the InfantRisk Center. Clinicians should consider the following when prescribing medications during lactation (**Box 3**).

Substance use

As previous stated, women who are using illicit drugs, for example, cocaine and phencyclidine, should not breastfeed.[73] Women who are stable on their opioid agonists should be encouraged to breastfeed.[73] Breastfeeding may help decrease the severity and duration of neonatal abstinence syndrome. Breastfeeding women should additionally be encouraged to cut down or stop using marijuana, as there is insufficient data to evaluate the effects of marijuana exposure via breastfeeding.[74] Tobacco use should be avoided to minimize harmful effects, and resources to stop should be provided; however, for women who are unable to stop smoking, outcomes of breastfed infants are better than outcomes of formula-fed infants. Alcohol intake should be infrequent; after consuming a single serving (12 oz of 5% beer, or 5 oz of 11% wine, or 1.5 oz of 40% liquor), women should avoid breastfeeding for at least 2 hours.[75] As alcohol

---

Box 3
Factors to consider when prescribing medications during lactation

- Maternal need for the medication.
- Potential effects of the drug on milk production.
- Amount of the drug excreted into human milk.
- Extent of oral absorption by the breastfeeding infant.
- Potential adverse effects on the breastfeeding infant.
- Age of the infant.
- Proportion of feedings that are breast milk.

Adapted from Centers for Disease Control and Prevention (CDC). Breastfeeding and Special Circumstances. Vaccinations, Medications, & Drugs. Prescription Medication Use. Available at: https://www.cdc.gov/breastfeeding/breastfeeding-special-circumstances/vaccinations-medications-drugs/prescription-medication-use.html. Accessed Dec 13 2019.

is cleared from the maternal circulation, it leaves the milk compartment by passive diffusion; thus, women do not need to express and discard milk after consuming a single serving of alcohol.

Social Challenges

Substantial inequities exist in breastfeeding initiation and duration by race and ethnicity. Among infants born in 2016, 86.6% of non-Hispanic White infants were ever breastfed, compared with 74.0% of non-Hispanic Black infants.[21] Breastfeeding initiation rates were lower among women with less education, who were younger, who had lower household incomes, or who were unmarried.

Addressing these inequities requires attention to structural determinants of health, including access to paid parental leave. The United States is the only high-income country in the world without any provision for paid parental leave. Although the Family and Medical Leave Act (FMLA) provides unpaid job-protected leave, it only covers a subset of workers and many cannot afford to go without pay for 3 months. As a result, in 2012, 23% of working women returned to the workplace within 10 days of giving birth.[76] Not surprisingly, paid leave increases breastfeeding rates: after California enacted paid leave in 2004, breastfeeding rates at 6 months increased 17.4%.[77] As of August 2019, 8 US states and the District of Columbia have enacted paid family and medical leave insurance.[78] Obstetric care providers should ensure that patients are aware of their rights under FMLA and are informed of any state paid leave provisions.

Reducing inequities also requires health care providers to confront our implicit biases. An integrative literature review found that African American women received inadequate or inaccurate information about breastfeeding from maternity care providers.[79] Asking open-ended questions, such as "What have you heard about infant feeding?" can center discussions on the patient's needs and understanding, rather than on the assumptions of the provider. Office practices and hospitals should also assess the extent to which photographs and posters include images of breastfeeding women that are congruent with their patient population. Stratifying quality metrics by race can further identify inequities in process measures that may aggravate disparities.

Return to Work

The "Break Time for Nursing Mothers" law requires employers to allow unpaid break time for employees to express milk for nursing children up to 1 year post partum in a private space that is not a bathroom.[80] However, 60% of women report that they do not have the time and space they need to express milk at work.[81] The Office of Women's Health provides detailed information for employers on how to support nursing mothers in the workplace.[82] It can be helpful to share this information with women during the prenatal period so that they can plan ahead with their employer and be prepared to express milk when they return to work. The Center for WorkLife Law provides a sample letter for maternity care providers to advocate for appropriate accommodations.[83]

SUMMARY

Breastfeeding provides medical and nonmedical benefits with few contraindications. Obstetric care providers can enable mothers to breastfeed by educating on the benefits of lactation, providing anticipatory guidance and practical breastfeeding support, understanding lactation physiology, building skills to manage common complications of lactation, and supporting policies that empower mothers to breastfeed and decrease infant feeding disparities.

DISCLOSURE

Society for Maternal Fetal Medicine Foundation Training Grant.

REFERENCES

1. Eidelman AI, Schanler RJ, Johnston M, et al. Breastfeeding and the use of human milk. Pediatrics 2012;129(3):e827–41.
2. IpS., Chung M, Raman G, et al. Breastfeeding and maternal and child health outcomes in developed countries.AHRQ Publication No 07-E007, 2007.
3. Bartick MC, Schwarz EB, Green BD, et al. Suboptimal breastfeeding in the United States: Maternal and pediatric health outcomes and costs. Matern Child Nutr 2016;13(1). https://doi.org/10.1111/mcn.12366.
4. Groer MW, Kendall-Tacket K. Clinics in human lactation: how breastfeeding protects women's health throughout the lifespan. The psychoneuroimmunology of human lactation. Amarillo(TX): Hale Publishing; 2011.
5. American College of Obstetricians and Gynecologists, ACOG Committee Opinion No. 756: Optimizing Support for Breastfeeding as Part of Obstetric Practice. ObstetGynecol 2018;132(4):e187–96.
6. Saxton A, Fahy K, Rolfe M, et al. Does skin-to-skin contact and breast feeding at birth affect the rate of primary postpartum haemorrhage: Results of a cohort study. Midwifery 2015;31(11):1110–7.
7. Chowdhury R, Sinha B, Sankar MJ, et al. Breastfeeding and maternal health outcomes: a systematic review and meta-analysis. ActaPaediatr 2015;104(S467): 96–113.
8. Wouk K, Gottfredson NC, Tucker C, et al. Positive emotions during infant feeding and postpartum mental health. J WomensHealth(Larchmt) 2019;28(2):194–202.
9. Gunderson EP, Jacobs DR Jr, Chiang V, et al. Duration of lactation and incidence of the metabolic syndrome in women of reproductive age according to gestational diabetes mellitus status: a 20-Year prospective study in CARDIA (Coronary Artery Risk Development in Young Adults). Diabetes 2010;59(2):495–504.
10. Ram KT, Bobby P, Hailpern SM, et al. Duration of lactation is associated with lower prevalence of the metabolic syndrome in midlife–SWAN, the study of women's health across the nation. Am J ObstetGynecol 2008;198(3):268.e1–6.
11. Feltner, C, Weber, R. Stuebe, A. et al., Breastfeeding Programs and Policies, Breastfeeding Uptake, and Maternal Health Outcomes in Developed Countries. Comparative Effectiveness Review No. 210. (Prepared by the RTI International– University of North Carolina at Chapel Hill Evidence-based Practice Center under Contract No. 290-2015-00011-I.) AHRQ Publication No. 18-EHC014-EF. Rockville, MD: Agency for Healthcare Research and Quality; July 2018. Posted final reports are located on the Effective Health Care Program search page. DOI:, Rockville (MD).
12. Jordan SJ, Na R, Johnatty SE, et al. Breastfeeding and endometrial cancer risk: an analysis from the epidemiology of endometrial cancer consortium. ObstetGynecol 2017;129(6):1059–67.
13. Yi X, Zhu J, Zhu X, et al. Breastfeeding and thyroid cancer risk in women: A dose-response meta-analysis of epidemiological studies. ClinNutr 2016;35(5):1039–46.
14. Committee Opinion No. 658: Optimizing Support for Breastfeeding as Part of Obstetric Practice. ObstetGynecol 2016;127(2):e86–92.

15. Vohr BR, Poindexter BB, Dusick AM, et al. Persistent beneficial effects of breast milk ingested in the neonatal intensive care unit on outcomes of extremely low birth weight infants at 30 months of age. Pediatrics 2007;120(4):e953–9.

16. Karlsson JO, Garnett T, Rollins NC, et al. The carbon footprint of breastmilk substitutes in comparison with breastfeeding. J Clean Prod 2019;222:436–45.

17. Joffe N, Webster F, Shenker N. Support for breastfeeding is an environmental imperative. BMJ 2019;367:l5646.

18. Stuebe AM. Does breastfeeding prevent the metabolic syndrome, or does the metabolic syndrome prevent breastfeeding? SeminPerinatol 2015;39(4):290–5.

19. World Health Organization, UNICEF. Global strategy for infant and young child feeding. Geneva: World Health Organization; 2003.

20. Centers for Disease Control and Prevention. Contraindications to breastfeeding or feeding expressed breast milk to infants. 2018. Available at:https://www.cdc.gov/breastfeeding/breastfeeding-special-circumstances/contraindications-to-breastfeeding.html. . Accessed December 14, 2019.

21. Centers for Disease Control and Prevention. Breastfeeding among U.S. Children born 2000-2016, CDC national Immunization survey. 2019. Available at:https://www.cdc.gov/breastfeeding/data/nis_data/results.html. . Accessed December 1, 2019.

22. Centers for Disease Control and Prevention. Maternal, infant, and child health 2010. 2016. Available at:https://www.healthypeople.gov/2020/topics-objectives/topic/maternal-infant-and-child-health/objectives. . Accessed October 1, 2016.

23. Centers for Disease Control and Prevention. Rates of any and exclusive breastfeeding by Socio-demographics among children born in 2016. 2019. Available at:https://www.cdc.gov/breastfeeding/data/nis_data/rates-any-exclusive-bf-socio-dem-2016.htm. . Accessed December 14, 2019.

24. Centers for Disease Control and Prevention. Progress in increasing breastfeeding and reducing racial/ethnic differences-United States, 2000-2008 births. MMWRMorb Mortal Wkly Rep 2013;62(5):77.

25. Louis-Jacques A, Deubel TF, Taylor M, et al. Racial and ethnic disparities in U.S. breastfeeding and implications for maternal and child health outcomes. SeminPerinatol 2017;41(5):299–307.

26. Bartick MC, Jegier BJ, Green BD, et al. Disparities in Breastfeeding: Impact on Maternal and Child Health Outcomes and Costs. J Pediatr 2017;181:49–55.e6.

27. Odom EC, Li R, Scanlon KS, et al. Reasons for earlier than desired cessation of breastfeeding. Pediatrics 2013;131(3):e726–32.

28. Stuebe AM, Horton BJ, Chetwynd E, et al. Prevalence and risk factors for early, undesired weaning attributed to lactation dysfunction. J WomensHealth(Larchmt) 2014;23(5):404–12.

29. Freed GL, Clark SJ, Cefalo RC, et al. Breast-feeding education of obstetrics-gynecology residents and practitioners. Am J ObstetGynecol 1995;173(5):1607–13.

30. Howard CR, Schaffer SJ, Lawrence RA. Attitudes, practices, and recommendations by obstetricians about infant feeding. Birth 1997;24(4):240–6.

31. Archabald K, Lundsberg L, Triche E, et al. Women's prenatal concerns regarding breastfeeding: are they being addressed? J MidwiferyWomensHealth 2011;56(1):2–7.

32. Cattaneo A, Buzzetti R. Effect on rates of breast feeding of training for the baby friendly hospital initiative. BMJ 2001;323(7325):1358–62.

33. Qureshy E, Louis-Jacques AF, Abunamous Y, et al. Impact of a formal lactation curriculum for residents on breastfeeding rates among low-income women. J Perinat Educ 2020;29(2):83–9.

34. Pang WW, Hartmann PE. Initiation of human lactation: secretory differentiation and secretory activation. J MammaryGlandBiolNeoplasia 2007;12(4):211–21.

35. Stuebe AM. Enabling women to achieve their breastfeeding goals. ObstetGynecol 2014;123(3):643–52.

36. Schanler RJ, Krebs NF, Mass SB, et al. Breastfeeding handbook for physicians. Chapter 5, Edition 2. American Academy of Pediatrics; 2013.

37. Rosen-Carole C, Hartman S, Academy of Breastfeeding Medicine. ABM Clinical Protocol #19: Breastfeeding Promotion in the Prenatal Setting, Revision 2015. Breastfeed Med 2015;10(10):451–7.

38. American College of Obstetricians and Gynecologists. Breastfeeding Toolkit. 2016.

39. Dewey KG, Nommsen-Rivers LA, Heinig MJ, et al. Risk factors for suboptimal infant breastfeeding behavior, delayed onset of lactation, and excess neonatal weight loss. Pediatrics 2003;112(3 Pt 1):607–19.

40. Beake S, Bick D, Narracott C, et al. Interventions for women who have a caesarean birth to increase uptake and duration of breastfeeding: A systematic review. Matern Child Nutr 2017;13(4). https://doi.org/10.1111/mcn.12390.

41. Moore ER, Bergman N, Anderson GC, et al. Early skin-to-skin contact for mothers and their healthy newborn infants. CochraneDatabaseSyst Rev 2016;(11):CD003519.

42. Bergman NJ. Neonatal stomach volume and physiology suggest feeding at 1-h intervals. ActaPaediatr 2013;102(8):773–7.

43. World Health Organization. Implementation guidance: protecting, promoting and supporting breastfeeding in facilities providing maternity and newborn services: the revised baby-friendly hospital initiative. 2018.

44. Ahrens KA, Hutcheon JA, Ananth CV, et al. Report of the office of population affairs' expert work group meeting on short birth spacing and adverse pregnancy outcomes: methodological quality of existing studies and future directions for research. PaediatrPerinatEpidemiol 2018;33(1):O5–14.

45. World Health Organization. Medical eligibility criteria for contraceptive use. Geneva (Switzerland): World Health Organization; 2015.

46. Centers for Disease Control and Prevention, U.S. Medical Eligibility Criteria for Contraceptive Use, 2016, in MMWRRecomm Rep. 2016, CDC: Atlanta, GA.

47. Kennedy KI, Rivera R, McNeilly AS. Consensus statement on the use of breastfeeding as a family planning method. Contraception 1989;39(5):477–96.

48. Mohammad MA, Hadsell DL, Haymond MW. Gene regulation of UDP-galactose synthesis and transport: potential rate-limiting processes in initiation of milk production in humans. Am J PhysiolEndocrinolMetab 2012;303(3):E365–76.

49. Phillips SJ, Tepper NK, Kapp N, et al. Progestogen-only contraceptive use among breastfeeding women: a systematic review. Contraception 2016;94(3):226–52.

50. Bryant AG, Lyerly AD, DeVane-Johnson S, et al. Hormonal contraception, breastfeeding, and bedside advocacy: the case for patient-centered care. Contraception 2019;99(2):73–6.

51. Tully KP, Stuebe AM, Verbiest SB. The 4th trimester: a critical transition period with unmet maternal health needs. Am J ObstetGynecol 2017;217(1):37–41. https://doi.org/10.1016/j.ajog.2017.03.032.

52. American College of Obstetricians and Gynecologists, ACOG Committee Opinion No. 736: Optimizing Postpartum Care. ObstetGynecol 2018;131(5): e140–50.

53. Trevathan W, Rosenberg KR. Costly and cute : helpless infants and human evolution. Santa Fe (NM): School for Advanced Research Press; 2016. Albuquerque : University of New Mexico Press, 2016.

54. Mangesi L, Dowswell T. Treatments for breast engorgement during lactation. Cochrane Database Syst Rev 2010;(9):CD006946.

55. Berens P, Brodribb W. ABM Clinical Protocol #20: Engorgement, Revised 2016. Breastfeed Med 2016;11(4):159–63.

56. Breastfeeding Medicine of Northeast Ohio. The basics of breast massage and hand expression. Available at: https://player.vimeo.com/video/65196007. Accsessed December 16 2019.

57. Berens P, Eglash A, Malloy M, et al. ABM Clinical Protocol #26: Persistent Pain with Breastfeeding. Breastfeed Med 2016;11(2):46–53.

58. Kellams A, Harrel C, Omage S, et al. ABM Clinical Protocol #3: Supplementary Feedings in the Healthy Term Breastfed Neonate, Revised 2017. Breastfeed Med 2017;12(4):188–98.

59. Neifert MR. Prevention of breastfeeding tragedies. PediatrClin North Am 2001; 48(2):273–97.

60. Evans A, Marinelli KA, Taylor JS. ABM clinical protocol #2: Guidelines for hospital discharge of the breastfeeding term newborn and mother: "The going home protocol," revised 2014. Breastfeed Med 2014;9(1):3–8.

61. Academy Of Breastfeeding Medicine Protocol Committee. ABM clinical protocol# 9: use of galactogogues in initiating or augmenting the rate of maternal milk secretion (First revision January 2011). Breastfeed Med 2011;6(1):41–9.

62. Grzeskowiak LE, Wlodek ME, Geddes DT. What evidence do we have for pharmaceutical galactagogues in the treatment of lactation insufficiency?-a narrative review. Nutrients 2019;11(5) [pii:E974].

63. Taylor A, Logan G, Twells L, et al. Human milk expression after domperidone treatment in postpartum women: a systematic review and meta-analysis of randomized controlled trials. J Hum Lact 2019;35(3):501–9.

64. Hale TW, Kendall-Tackett K, Cong Z. Domperidone versus metoclopramide: self-reported side effects in a large sample of breastfeeding mothers who used these medications to increase milk production. Clin Lactation 2018;9(1):10–7. https://doi.org/10.1891/2158-0782.9.1.10.

65. Nommsen-Rivers L, Thompson A, Riddle S, et al. Feasibility and acceptability of metformin to augment low milk supply: a pilot randomized controlled trial. J Hum Lact 2019;35(2):261–71.

66. Amir LH, Academy of Breastfeeding Medicine Protocol Committee. ABM Clinical Protocol #4: Mastitis, Revised March 2014. Breastfeed Med 2014;9(5):239–43.

67. Sisk PM, Lovelady CA, Dillard RG, et al. Lactation counseling for mothers of very low birth weight infants: effect on maternal anxiety and infant intake of human milk. Pediatrics 2006;117(1):e67–75.

68. Furman L, Minich N, Hack MJP. Correlates of lactation in mothers of very low birth weight infants. Pediatrics 2002;109(4):e57.

69. Parker L, Sullivan S, Krueger C, et al. Effect of early breast milk expression on milk volume and timing of lactogenesis stage II among mothers of very low birth weight infants: a pilot study. J Perinatol 2012;32(3):205.

70. Morton J, Hall J, Wong R, et al. Combining hand techniques with electric pumping increases milk production in mothers of preterm infants. J Perinatol 2009; 29(11):757.
71. Spiesser-Robelet L, Brunie V, de Andrade V, et al. Knowledge, representations, attitudes, and behaviors of women faced with taking medications while breastfeeding: A scoping review. J Hum Lact 2017;33(1):98–114.
72. Hussainy SY, Dermele N. Knowledge, attitudes and practices of health professionals and women towards medication use in breastfeeding: A review. Int Breastfeed J 2011;6(1):11.
73. Reece-Stremtan S, Marinelli KA, Medicine AoB. ABM clinical protocol# 21: guidelines for breastfeeding and substance use or substance use disorder, revised 2015. Breastfeed Med 2015;10(3):135–41.
74. Metz TD, Borgelt LM. Marijuana Use in Pregnancy and While Breastfeeding. ObstetGynecol 2018;132(5):1198–210.
75. Koren G. Drinking alcohol while breastfeeding. Will it harm my baby? Can FamPhysician 2002;48:39–41.
76. Klerman JA, Daley K, Pozniak A. Family and medical leave in 2012: technical report 2014. Cambridg (MA).
77. Huang R, Yang M. Paid maternity leave and breastfeeding practice before and after California's implementation of the nation's first paid family leave program. Econ Hum Biol 2015;16:45–59.
78. National partnership for women & families. State paid family and medical leave Insurance laws, August 2019. 2019. Available at: https://www.nationalpartnership. org/our-work/resources/economic-justice/paid-leave/state-paid-family-leave-laws. pdf. Accessed December 1, 2019.
79. DeVane-Johnson S, Woods-Giscombe C, Thoyre S, et al. Integrative Literature Review of Factors Related to Breastfeeding in African American Women: Evidence for a Potential Paradigm Shift. J Hum Lact 2017;33(2):435–47.
80. U.S. Department of Labor. Fact Sheet #73: break time for nursing mothers under the FLSA. 2019. Available at:https://www.dol.gov/whd/regs/compliance/whdfs73. htm. . Accessed December 1, 2019.
81. Kozhimannil KB, Jou J, Gjerdingen DK, et al. Access to workplace accommodations to support breastfeeding after passage of the affordable care act. Womens Health Issues 2016;26(1):6–13.
82. Office of Women's Health. Support nursing moms at work. 2019. Available at:https:// www.womenshealth.gov/supporting-nursing-moms-work. . Accessed December 1, 2019.
83. Pregnant@Work. Helping patients seek breastfeeding accomodations. 2019. Available at: https://www.pregnantatwork.org/healthcare-professionals/breastfeeding/. Accessed December 1, 2019.

Gestational Diabetes
Importance of Follow-up Screening for the Benefit of Long-term Health

Sydney M. Thayer, MD[a],*, Jamie O. Lo, MD[a],
Aaron B. Caughey, MD, PhD[a]

KEYWORDS

- Gestational diabetes • Postpartum glucose testing • Glucose intolerance
- Insulin resistance

KEY POINTS

- Gestational diabetes mellitus (GDM) is the most common obstetric metabolic disorder.
- Multiple long-term health outcomes have been associated with GDM, including type 2 diabetes, metabolic syndrome, and cardiovascular disease.
- Postpartum glucose screening is recommended following a GDM pregnancy for early identification of persistent hyperglycemia and to engage patients in chronic disease prevention.
- Rates of postpartum diabetes screening are poor. Barriers to screening include patient fears, provider misconceptions, and poor coordination of patient transition out of obstetric care.
- Interventions to increase screening rates are underway, including reminder systems and individualized education on chronic disease prevention, such that early risk identification and chronic disease prevention can be achieved.

INTRODUCTION

Gestational diabetes mellitus (GDM), or glucose intolerance in pregnancy, is the most common obstetrics metabolic disorder, with 3% to 14% of pregnancies complicated by GDM.[1,2] Poor antepartum and intrapartum glucose control is associated with many adverse neonatal outcomes, including shoulder dystocia, macrosomia, neonatal hypoglycemia, and stillbirth.[3] As such, a significant clinical emphasis is placed on the timely diagnosis, tight glucose control, and antenatal surveillance of women with GDM.

[a] Department of Obstetrics and Gynecology, Oregon Health and Science University, 3181 Southwest Sam Jackson Park Road, Portland, OR 97239, USA
* Corresponding author.
E-mail address: thayers@ohsu.edu

The long-term health outcomes in women with a history of GDM is a topic of great interest. Type 2 diabetes mellitus (T2DM), metabolic syndrome, and cardiovascular disease are commonly reported associations with GDM.[1,4,5] The early primary goal of detecting GDM through glucose intolerance screening was to predict the risk of later development of T2DM. Women with a GDM history have a 25% incidence of metabolic syndrome within 5 years postpartum, as well as a 70% chance of progressing to T2DM and a 2.3-fold increased risk of cardiovascular disease in the 10 years postpartum.[6–8] Although interventions are available to decrease the risk of these long-term health outcomes, many practitioners lack the resources to systematically identify women who would benefit most from such targeted chronic disease prevention measures.[9,10]

Given the risk of adverse long-term health outcomes, postpartum glucose screening is recommended for women with a prior pregnancy complicated by GDM. Although multiple professional societies agree on the utility and recommendation for postpartum glucose screening, low patient compliance persists.[3,11–14] Contributors to poor screening rates include patient fears, provider misconceptions, confusion regarding guideline variations, and barriers to reliable health care transitions. Interventions to increase postpartum screening uptake range from patient reminder systems to establishing consistent health care communication channels, including emphasizing provider education on the associations between GDM and future chronic diseases .

Women are often motivated to make positive health decisions during pregnancy, making this engaged population an important target for enacting lifelong health care changes. Obstetrics and primary care providers have a unique role in educating women regarding the adverse health outcomes associated with GDM and the recommended postpartum screening. These measures are an opportunity for early identification, intervention, and prevention of potential future chronic disease in a population of young women that may otherwise be unrecognized until later in life.

DIAGNOSIS OF GESTATIONAL DIABETES MELLITUS AND POSTPARTUM HYPERGLYCEMIA
Gestational Diabetes

Gestational diabetes is defined as glucose intolerance diagnosed for the first time in pregnancy that is not clearly overt diabetes.[3] Glucose intolerance is a measure traditionally defined by the response to an oral glucose challenge conducted routinely at 24 to 28 weeks of pregnancy.[3] Historically, GDM diagnosis involved a 2 step approach consisting of a screening 1-hour 50-g glucose challenge followed by a confirmatory 3-hour 100-g oral glucose tolerance test (OGTT). A 1-hour result of greater than or equal to 140 mg/dL (7.8 mmol/L) is considered an abnormal screening value. The original diagnostic criteria recommended by the National Diabetes Data Group (NDDG) were based on the results of O'Sullivan and Mahan,[15] but in 1982 the criteria were amended to be more inclusive in response to newer findings by Carpenter and Coustan.[16] As the prevalence of GDM increased and additional research findings were reported, the need for updated consensus guidelines grew. In 2007, the Fifth International Workshop-Conference on Gestational Diabetes recommended diagnostic criteria for GDM based on the 100-g oGTT, in which 2 or more for the following glucose values must be abnormal to obtain the diagnosis - fasting 95-125 mg/dL, 1 hour >/= 190 mg/dL, 2 hour >/= 165, and 3 hour >/= 145.[17] The diagnostic recommendations were further modified following the Hyperglycemic and Adverse Pregnancy Outcomes (HAPO) study in 2008, which showed increased rates of fetal and maternal adverse effects with increasing hyperglycemia.[18] In response to these results, the International Association of the Diabetes and Pregnancy Study Groups (IADPSG) outlined new diagnostic criteria in 2010 to lower the numeric threshold for the diagnosis of GDM, which were adopted by the World Health Organization (WHO) in 2013 and the American Diabetes Association (ADA) in 2014.[19–21] The HAPO results focused on a 1 step approach consisting of a single 75-g OGTT to define GDM. With this test, gestational diabetes is diagnosed if, at any point during gestation, 1 or more of the criteria in **Table 1** are met.[20] The National Institutes of Health maintains the recommendation for a 2-step diagnostic approach in the United States until stronger, prospective evidence is available to support the IADPSG threshold changes. Alternatively, the diagnosis of overt diabetes is made if, at any time (either during or outside of pregnancy), the criteria in **Table 2** are met in the presence of classic diabetic symptoms (excessive thirst, frequent urination, unintentional weight loss), or if a random plasma glucose level is greater than or equal to 200 mg/dL (11.1 mmol/L) in the presence of diabetic symptoms.[20]

Postpartum Glucose Intolerance

The ADA recommends glucose intolerance testing at 4 to 12 weeks postpartum using a 2-hour 75-g OGTT.[3] Hyperglycemia not meeting criteria for overt diabetes (see **Table 2**) is defined by impaired fasting glucose (IFG) level or impaired glucose tolerance (IGT). IFG is regarded as fasting plasma glucose (FPG) 100 to 125 mg/dL (5.6–6.9 mmol/L).[22] Using the 75-g OGTT, IGT is classified as a 2-hour value of 140 to 199 mg/dL (7.8–11.0 mmol/L).[22]

INCIDENCE OF GESTATIONAL DIABETES MELLITUS AND POSTPARTUM GLUCOSE INTOLERANCE

Gestational diabetes is diagnosed in 3% to 14% of pregnant women, with 1 in 4 pregnancies complicated by some degree of hyperglycemia.[1,12] The increasing prevalence of gestational glucose intolerance is partly caused by the obesity epidemic.[23] In the United States, the incidence of GDM is highest among women of African American, Native American, Pacific Islander, Hispanic American, and South or East Asian ethnic groups.[24–26] Although the GDM population is highly heterogeneous, women with GDM may be grouped according to their insulin sensitivity and insulin secretion profiles.[27] Half of women with GDM are primarily insulin resistant, 30% have primarily impaired insulin secretion, and the remaining 20% have a combination of both.[27]

The incidence of isolated postpartum IFG is 3% to 6% among women tested, but the incidence of IGT can range from 7% to 29% at 4 to 20 weeks postpartum.[28] Postpartum diagnosis of overt diabetes is identified in 5% to 14% of women who received treatment of GDM during pregnancy.[28]

Table 1	
Diagnostic criteria for 75-g oral glucose tolerance test for gestational diabetes	
Examination Interval (h)	**Plasma Glucose Concentration**
Fasting	5.1–6.9 mmol/L (92–125 mg/dL)
1	≥10.0 mmol/L (153–199 mg/dL)
2	8.5–11.0 mmol/L (153–199 mg/dL)

Adapted from Diagnostic criteria and classification of hyperglycaemia first detected in pregnancy: A World Health Organization Guideline. Diabetes Res Clin Pract 2014;103(3):341-363; with permission.

Table 2	
Diagnostic criteria for overt diabetes	
Examination Interval (h)	**Plasma Glucose Concentration**
Fasting	≥126 mg/dL (≥7.0 mmol/L)
2	≥200 mg/dL (≥11.1 mmol/L)

Adapted from Diagnostic criteria and classification of hyperglycaemia first detected in pregnancy: A World Health Organization Guideline. Diabetes Res Clin Pract 2014;103(3):341-363; with permission.

POSTPARTUM GLUCOSE INTOLERANCE TESTING AND ADVERSE LONG-TERM HEALTH OUTCOMES ASSOCIATED WITH GESTATIONAL DIABETES MELLITUS

Early postpartum identification of women with IGT can decrease long-term adverse health events in women with a prior GDM pregnancy through risk modification and primary prevention. However, persistent hyperglycemia diagnostic of T2DM in the immediate postpartum period (within 1–3 days) is uncommon. Thus, delayed glucose testing is recommended until 4 to 12 weeks postpartum when IGT is detected in 17% to 23% of women with antecedent GDM pregnancies.[28]

Early recognition of postpartum IFG or IGT identifies women at risk of future medical complications. Compared to those with normoglycemic pregnancies, women with GDM have greater than 7-times increased lifetime risk of T2DM; 60% of women with GDM develop T2DM within 10 years postpartum.[7,10] Women with an abnormal 2-hour plasma glucose concentration on OGTT have increased rates of conversion to T2DM within 6 months postpartum as opposed to 5 years.[29] Thus, failure to obtain follow-up diabetes screening after childbirth may have significant implications, including patient presentation to care with acute symptoms or chronic disease exacerbations caused by the lack of early diabetes management.

Further, women with undiagnosed IGT postpartum have increased risk of entering a subsequent pregnancy with hyperglycemia, which may affect both maternal and fetal health. Bernstein and colleagues[30] found that those with GDM who had a subsequent term live birth within 3 years of the index pregnancy had a GDM recurrence rate of 49.3% regardless of the interval to next conception. In addition, women with another GDM pregnancy have 3 times the odds of early-onset T2DM within 3 years of the second delivery.[30] Shorter interpregnancy interval (≤1 year vs 3 years) further increases lifetime risk of T2DM, increasing the likelihood of entering a pregnancy with IGT caused by unrecognized postpartum hyperglycemia.[30]

Progression to Type 2 Diabetes Mellitus

T2DM is a common long-term health outcome in women with a history of GDM. Within 5 years of a GDM pregnancy, 20% to 50% of women progress to T2DM, with up to 70% developing T2DM within 10 years.[1,7] A recent large meta-analysis of 2.6 million women showed that those with GDM have an odds ratio (OR) of 17.9 of developing T2DM.[31] Another large systematic review reported a 7-fold increased risk of T2DM in women with a history of GDM.[7]

The progression to T2DM is partly attributed to decreased insulin sensitivity and impaired beta-cell compensation in women with a history of GDM.[32] The degree of glucose intolerance during pregnancy may be predictive of future T2DM.[33] Women treated with insulin or oral glycemic medications during pregnancy have increased rates of T2DM at 6 to 9 weeks postpartum compared with those with diet-controlled GDM.[33] Bernstein and colleagues[30] showed an adjusted OR (aOR) of

2.36 for T2DM when comparing women with medication-controlled GDM with women who were diet controlled.

Multiple factors are associated with future diagnosis of T2DM, including an earlier gestational age (<24 weeks) at GDM diagnosis, higher fasting blood glucose level, frequent insulin use, advanced maternal age, nonwhite ethnicity, family history of diabetes, and recurrence of GDM in a subsequent pregnancy.[30,34,35] Obesity, defined by prepregnancy body mass index (BMI) greater than 30 kg/m^2, further increases the risk of T2DM within 5 years postpartum.[29,35] These factors have been used in risk assessment scores for predicting the development of T2DM after GDM. **Table 3** shows the clinical calculation proposed by Köhler and colleagues[36] for T2DM risk during the 5 years following a GDM pregnancy, with less than or equal to 140 total points conferring an 11% risk, 141 to 220 a 29% risk, 221 to 300 a 64% risk, and greater than 300 suggestive of an 80% risk of developing T2DM.

Metabolic Syndrome

Gestational diabetes is associated with hypertension, dyslipidemia, and vascular dysfunction, as well as central obesity and insulin resistance.[5] These clinical comorbidities are characteristic of metabolic syndrome, a condition more precisely defined for female patients by the International Diabetes Federation (IDF) and the National Cholesterol Education Program (NCEP) Adult Treatment Panel III (ATPIII) in **Table 4**.[37,38]

Women with a history of GDM have increased odds of central obesity (OR, 2.64), hypertriglyceridemia (OR, 3.68–4.14), hyperglycemia (OR, 1.62), and hypertension (OR, 3.60).[4,39,40] In a previous Danish study, women with a history of diet-controlled GDM were 3 times more likely to develop metabolic syndrome than age-matched controls.[41] Huvinen and colleagues[6] found that, among women with a GDM history, 25% are diagnosed with metabolic syndrome by 5 years postpartum, but the incidence in obese women with the same history is even higher at 39%. Further, women with increased body fat percentage and a history of GDM have an aOR of 3.66 to 3.90 for developing metabolic syndrome, which is higher than those without GDM.[4]

Cardiovascular Health

Women with a history of GDM are at increased risk for deleterious cardiovascular outcomes including hypertension, stroke, and myocardial ischemia.[5,42] The cause of this risk may be increased levels of inflammatory markers, which can result in atherosclerosis and future adverse events.[32] In a prospective study of nearly 90,000 women in the United States over the age of 26 years, those with a GDM history had a 43% greater risk of cerebrovascular disease compared with women without prior GDM.[5]

Table 3	
Type 2 diabetes mellitus risk assessment calculator	
Risk Factor	**Points Allotted**
BMI	5 × BMI (kg/m^2)
GDM treated with insulin	+132
Family history of diabetes	+44
Breastfed infant	−35

From Köhler M, Ziegler AG, Beyerlein A. Development of a simple tool to predict the risk of postpartum diabetes in women with gestational diabetes mellitus. Acta Diabetol 2016;53(3):433-437; with permission.

Table 4
Metabolic disorder definitions

	IDF	NCEP ATPIII
Definition	Central obesity + at least 2 additional criteria:	At least 3 of the following:
Central Obesity	Waist circumference ≥80 cm	Waist circumference ≥80 cm
Triglyceride Levels	>150 mg/dL or using specific treatment of lipid abnormalities	>150 mg/dL or using specific treatment of lipid abnormalities
HDL Cholesterol Level	<50 mg/dL or using specific treatment of this lipid abnormality	—
Blood Pressure	SBP ≥ 130 mm Hg or DBP ≥ 85 mm Hg or using antihypertensive agent	SBP ≥ 130 mm Hg or DBP ≥ 85 mm Hg or using antihypertensive agent
FPG Level	>100 mg/dL or previously diagnosed T2DM	>100 mg/dL or using agent for treatment of increased glucose level

Abbreviations: DBP, diastolic blood pressure; HDL, high-density lipoprotein; SBP, systolic blood pressure.

Adapted from Alberti KG, Zimmet P, Shaw J, et al. The metabolic syndrome–a new worldwide definition. Lancet 2005;366(9491):1060; and Grundy SM, Cleeman JI, Daniels SR, et al. Diagnosis and management of the metabolic syndrome: an American Heart Association/National Heart, Lung, and Blood Institute Scientific Statement. Circulation 2005;112(17):2739; with permission.

McKenzie-Sampson and colleagues[43] studied more than 1 million Canadian women with GDM and found higher rates of ischemic heart disease, myocardial infarction, coronary angioplasty, and coronary artery bypass grafting in the 25 years postpartum compared with those without a GDM history.[43] A meta-analysis that included almost 5.4 million women internationally reported that women with a history of GDM have a 2.3-fold increased risk of cardiovascular events in the decade after pregnancy compared to those without, independent of T2DM status.[8] These findings are alarming, because these women are often young and otherwise unlikely to experience a major cardiovascular event outside of their history of GDM.

INTERVENTIONS TO DECREASE THE RISK OF ADVERSE HEALTH OUTCOMES

Because of the well-established relationship between GDM and chronic diseases, identifying and implementing interventions to decrease the incidence of associated health complications is a priority. Breastfeeding has been found to be protective against obesity and glucose intolerance in postpartum women.[28] Postpartum healthy dietary intake and regular exercise have shown reduced progression to diabetes for women with a history of GDM, as well as lower risk of cardiovascular-related chronic disease including hypertension.[9,10,42,43] In the 10 years following an index GDM pregnancy, intensive lifestyle modifications and the use of metformin were found to reduce progression to T2DM by 35% and 40%, respectively, and the number needed to treat to prevent 1 case of T2DM in the 3 years postpartum is 5 to 6.[9,44]

RECOMMENDATIONS FOR POSTPARTUM GLUCOSE INTOLERANCE SCREENING

Multiple professional guidelines exist for postpartum diabetes testing in women with a history of GDM (**Table 5**), which largely recommend using a 2-hour OGTT

Table 5
Recommended guidelines for postpartum diabetes screening among women with gestational diabetes mellitus

Year	Organization	Postpartum Testing Period Recommended (wk)	Recommended Test
2007	Fifth International Workshop-Conference on Gestational Diabetes Mellitus	6–12	2-h 75-g OGTT[17]
2013	Endocrine Society	6–12	2-h 75-g OGTT[67]
2013	American College of Obstetricians and Gynecologists	6–12	2-h 75-g OGTT or FPG[11]
2015	National Institute for Health and Care Excellent	6–13	FPG[45]
2018	ADA	4–12	2-h 75-g OGTT[3]

with the diabetes criteria for nonpregnant individuals, as previously discussed. However, a few organizations recommend using FPG instead, given the relative ease and patient acceptance of performing the test postpartum. The National Institute for Health and Care Excellence (NIHCE) endorses offering FPG testing at 6 to 13 weeks postpartum.[45] Although NIHCE found that up to 40% more women would be diagnosed with T2DM using the 75-g OGTT compared with FPG alone, only up to 50% of women diagnosed with GDM completed their recommended OGTT postpartum.[45] Thus, the NIHCE recommends an abnormal screening FPG ($\geq$6.0 mmol/L) should be followed with a confirmatory test (second FPG, hemoglobin A1c [HbA1c], or 75-g 2-hour OGTT).[45] Thus, women who are reluctant to submit to the standard recommended diabetes testing may initially screen with fasting blood glucose; the reported value will alert the clinician to assess if further testing would be beneficial.

In women with a normal postpartum OGTT, the ADA recommends diabetes testing every 1 to 3 years thereafter using HbA1c, FPG, or a 2-hour 75-g OGTT with nonpregnant thresholds.[3] Testing frequency should depend on the woman's specific risk factors, including family history, prepregnancy BMI, and need for medical management to achieve glycemic control during pregnancy.[3] Women with increased postpartum glucose levels not diagnostic of diabetes should undergo annual testing, a recommendation echoed by NIHCE, which advises annual HbA1c testing for women diagnosed with GDM who have negative postnatal diabetes screening.[45]

POSTPARTUM GLUCOSE SCREENING
Patient Screening

Despite the broad recommendation for postpartum glucose screening, patient screening rates are overall low, with as few as 16% to 22.5% of women with GDM undergoing postpartum diabetes testing.[13,14,34] Shah and colleagues[13] showed that, despite 94% to 97% of women having ambulatory care visits in the 6 months postpartum, more than 60% of women with GDM had no diabetes testing and only 4.5% completed the recommended OGTT. Within a cohort of 1078 primarily black urban women in Missouri with GDM, only 8.4% of women fulfilled the recommended diabetes screening in the 4 to 12 weeks postpartum.[46] One year postpartum, the proportion of women undergoing screening increased to 18.9% for the 2-hour 75-g OGTT and 40.6% for any form of glucose testing.[46] In comparison, patients receiving care at academic centers showed greater compliance, but still with only 33.7% completing either FPG or 2-hour 75-g OGTT postpartum.[47] This finding suggests that at least two-thirds of women are not undergoing recommended postpartum diabetes testing.

Because of concern for low postpartum screening compliance, efforts are underway to increase the proportion of women tested for diabetes after a GDM pregnancy. These approaches have largely focused on examining and addressing the barriers to follow-up at the patient, provider, and systems levels, particularly when transitions in health care are involved.[48]

Factors Influencing Postpartum Screening

Although postpartum glucose screening is not optimally observed, factors associated with increased compliance include maternal age greater than or equal to 35 years, nulliparity, higher income, Asian-American ethnicity, and advanced educational degrees.[47,49] Women with insulin-treated GDM are more likely to follow up than women with diet-controlled GDM, and women with a history of GDM in more than 1 pregnancy are more adherent to postpartum screening guidelines.[47,50] Using integrated health care systems improves postpartum diabetes screening compliance, with some reporting rates as high as 60%.[24] In contrast, the challenges to postpartum screening are often found in the natural care transitions that occur following pregnancy.

Transition from pregnancy to postpartum
The initial barrier to patients completing postpartum glucose screening arises in the transition from pregnancy to postpartum care. Inconsistent screening recommendations from professional societies creates provider uncertainty surrounding the timing and choice of test and results in missed screening opportunities.[12] Further, there is a misperception among some providers and patients that women with GDM have a low risk of developing T2DM and thus less emphasis is placed on follow-up screening.[12,51–53] In addition, although focusing on the immediate fetal risk is a common and effective motivational tool, this approach may mislead women to assume postpartum testing is unnecessary because GDM is "cured" with delivery.[12,53] As such, as few as one-third of women with GDM identify themselves as having an increased risk of future diabetes.[51]

Patient factors and demographics also create barriers to screening. Castling and Farrell[54] found that 74% of women who failed to undergo recommended postpartum glucose testing were in the bottom 2 quintiles of socioeconomic status and have a higher likelihood of tobacco use, unemployment, and teen motherhood. The emotional stress of adjusting to motherhood and preoccupation with a new baby further contribute to decreased postpartum visit attendance.[12,34,52,55] Fear of a diabetes diagnosis and the need to fast before undergoing an OGTT are common reasons reported by women for avoiding postpartum testing.[34,52,53,56]

Transition from postpartum to primary care
The return to primary care is another transition where diabetes screening barriers arise. Incomplete communication between obstetrics and primary care providers results in decreased awareness of the patient's pregnancy complications and thus failure to perform necessary follow-up. It is often unclear which provider is responsible for scheduling testing, arranging clinical visits, and sending follow-up reminders;

thus, these responsibilities may be overlooked.[12,53] Further, as many as 40% of women with Medicaid insurance do not establish with a primary care provider post-partum, resulting in missed opportunities for disease screening and timely initiation of preventive treatments.[46,56] Even among women with GDM who undergo the initial recommended postpartum glucose screening, most have decreased testing rates in subsequent years.[57] This lack of long-term follow-up compliance may be secondary to the absence of patient-tracking and reminder systems for subsequent testing, incomplete patient hand-offs between prenatal and primary care providers, or the false reassurance of patient glucose normalization after delivery.[57,58] A prior study reported that women with GDM with normal postpartum glucose testing were significantly heavier 2 years after delivery than women who did not complete postpartum testing, suggesting that a false perception of health may lead to worse future outcomes.[58]

STRATEGIES TO INCREASE POSTPARTUM SCREENING

To address the barriers identified, multiple approaches have been suggested to increase postpartum glucose testing rates. During the antepartum and immediate postpartum periods, education should be provided that explicitly emphasizes the association of GDM with future chronic diseases. Women who perceive a high lifetime future risk of diabetes are more likely to make positive behavioral changes.[51] A 2008 study found that postpartum follow-up testing rates increased from 18% to 57% after initiating an antepartum education initiative highlighting the future health consequences linked with GDM.[59] Another study noted that, when nurse care-managers conducted at least 3 antepartum visits with women with GDM, there was increased awareness of potential long-term health outcomes and improved postpartum screening rates.[60] A single antepartum counseling visit by a nurse educator at 37 to 38 weeks increased rates of postpartum diabetes testing from 33% to 53%.[60] Adherence to postpartum follow-up is further improved by proactive systems, including personalized risk counseling for patients by providers.[12] Tailoring diabetes prevention strategies to a patient's health literacy level may also address demographic barriers.[61]

In the postpartum period, patient or provider reminder systems, such as telephone, text message, e-mail, and postal reminders, have been shown to increase rates of glucose tolerance testing.[52,62] Australia and Belgium have developed recall registries to send patient screening reminders for at least 5 years following a diagnosis of GDM and have shown improved rates of postpartum screening utilizing this method.[12] A randomized controlled study found that postpartum postal reminders for OGTT sent to patients, physicians, or both increased the rates of follow-up screening from 14.3% to 51% to 60%.[63]

In addition, establishing effective communication channels between obstetrics and primary care providers would better guarantee that women receive proper postpartum testing. Ensuring patients confirm a primary care provider before postpartum hospital discharge would promote a smoother transition from obstetric care.[53] Dedicated nurse coordinators who follow women with GDM in the postpartum period and provide personalized reminders until postpartum testing is completed can markedly increase adherence rates for postpartum screening; a study found that this intervention increased postpartum diabetes screening from 9% to more than 70%.[64] This is an example of a type of patient-centered home, in which systems are in place to provide continuity during transition points that would improve communication between maternity and primary care providers.[53]

POSTPARTUM SCREENING: FUTURE DIRECTIONS

Efforts to investigate other potential postpartum diabetes screening modalities for women with GDM are underway, including the use of HbA1c. However, pregnant women have increased turnover of erythrocytes, which causes HbA1c to underestimate the average glucose level in the bloodstream. This physiologic state persists to a degree in the postpartum period and has been the rationale for avoiding its use in postpartum diabetes screening. Although a prior meta-analysis found that HbA1c had a sensitivity of 36% for detecting postpartum diabetes, the utility of HbA1c in pregnancy and postpartum continues to be studied because of the convenience of performing the test in the nonfasting state.[65] Claesson and colleagues[66] evaluated the use of HbA1c in the third trimester to identify women at risk of diabetes postpartum and found that a HbA1c level of 5.7% to 6.4% identified women who would develop postpartum diabetes with 97% specificity and 91% positive predictive value, but the sensitivity was low. Thus, although not an effective screening tool to predict postpartum T2DM, HbA1c may identify high-risk women to target for lifestyle interventions. Allalou and colleagues[33] studied other biomarkers in women with GDM that develop T2DM and identified 21 metabolites that significantly differ in fasting plasma samples. These studies are currently in their infancy but may eventually guide risk stratification for women with GDM.

SUMMARY

Gestational diabetes increases a woman's lifetime risk of chronic diseases, including T2DM, metabolic syndrome, and cardiovascular disease. This pregnancy condition and its associated health complications will continue to be a significant public health concern without implementation of early and successful identification, intervention, and prevention strategies. An increased antenatal awareness of the potential long-term risks, as well as ensuring reliable follow-up and postpartum glucose testing, are important measures to address the current poor postpartum screening compliance. Emphasizing education of patients and providers about postpartum glucose screening is of utmost importance and has significant implications for long-term health.

DISCLOSURE

The authors have nothing to disclose.

REFERENCES

1. Kim C, Newton KM, Knopp RH. Gestational diabetes and the incidence of type 2 diabetes: a systematic review. Diabetes Care 2002;25(10):1862–8.
2. Correa A, Bardenheier B, Elixhauser A, et al. Trends in prevalence of diabetes among delivery hospitalizations, United States, 1993-2009. Matern Child Health J 2015;19(3):635–42.
3. American Diabetes Association. 14. Management of Diabetes in Pregnancy: Standards of Medical Care in Diabetes—2019. Diabetes Care 2019; 42(Supplement 1):S165–72.
4. Shen Y, Li W, Leng J, et al. High risk of metabolic syndrome after delivery in pregnancies complicated by gestational diabetes. Diabetes Res Clin Pract 2019;150: 219–26.

5. Tobias DK, Stuart JJ, Li S, et al. Association of History of Gestational Diabetes With Long-term Cardiovascular Disease Risk in a Large Prospective Cohort of US Women. JAMA Intern Med 2017;177(12):1735–42.

6. Huvinen E, Eriksson JG, Koivusalo SB, et al. Heterogeneity of gestational diabetes (GDM) and long-term risk of diabetes and metabolic syndrome: findings from the RADIEL study follow-up. Acta Diabetol 2018;55(5):493–501.

7. Bellamy L, Casas J-P, Hingorani AD, et al. Type 2 diabetes mellitus after gestational diabetes: a systematic review and meta-analysis. Lancet 2009;373(9677): 1773–9.

8. Kramer CK, Campbell S, Retnakaran R. Gestational diabetes and the risk of cardiovascular disease in women: a systematic review and meta-analysis. Diabetologia 2019;62(6):905–14.

9. Aroda VR, Christophi CA, Edelstein SL, et al. The effect of lifestyle intervention and metformin on preventing or delaying diabetes among women with and without gestational diabetes: the Diabetes Prevention Program outcomes study 10-year follow-up. J Clin Endocrinol Metab 2015;100(4):1646–53.

10. Tobias DK, Hu FB, Chavarro J, et al. Healthful dietary patterns and type 2 diabetes mellitus risk among women with a history of gestational diabetes mellitus. Arch Intern Med 2012;172(20):1566–72.

11. Committee on Practice Bulletins–Obstetrics. Practice Bulletin No. 137: Gestational diabetes mellitus. Obstet Gynecol 2013;122(2 Pt 1):406–16.

12. Balaji B, Ranjit Mohan A, Rajendra P, et al. Gestational Diabetes Mellitus Postpartum Follow-Up Testing: Challenges and Solutions. Can J Diabetes 2019. https://doi.org/10.1016/j.jcjd.2019.04.011.

13. Shah BR, Lipscombe LL, Feig DS, et al. Missed opportunities for type 2 diabetes testing following gestational diabetes: a population-based cohort study. BJOG 2011;118(12):1484–90.

14. Blatt AJ, Nakamoto JM, Kaufman HW. Gaps in diabetes screening during pregnancy and postpartum. Obstet Gynecol 2011;117(1):61–8.

15. O'sullivan JB, Mahan CM. Criteria for the oral glucose tolerance test in pregnancy. Diabetes 1964;13:278–85.

16. Carpenter MW, Coustan DR. Criteria for screening tests for gestational diabetes. Am J Obstet Gynecol 1982;144(7):768–73.

17. Metzger BE, Buchanan TA, Coustan DR, et al. Summary and Recommendations of the Fifth International Workshop-Conference on Gestational Diabetes Mellitus. Diabetes Care 2007;30(Supplement 2):S251–60.

18. HAPO Study Cooperative Research Group, Metzger BE, Lowe LP, Dyer AR, et al. Hyperglycemia and adverse pregnancy outcomes. N Engl J Med 2008;358(19): 1991–2002.

19. Metzger BE, Gabbe SG, Persson B, et al. International Association of Diabetes and Pregnancy Study Groups Recommendations on the Diagnosis and Classification of Hyperglycemia in Pregnancy: Response to Weinert. Diabetes Care 2010;33(7):e98.

20. Diagnostic criteria and classification of hyperglycaemia first detected in pregnancy: A World Health Organization Guideline. Diabetes Res Clin Pract 2014; 103(3):341–63.

21. American Diabetes Association. Standards of Medical Care in Diabetes—2014. Diabetes Care 2014;37(Supplement 1):S14–80.

22. American Diabetes Association. Diagnosis and Classification of Diabetes Mellitus. Diabetes Care 2014;37(Supplement 1):S81–90.

23. Kampmann U, Madsen LR, Skajaa GO, et al. Gestational diabetes: A clinical update. World J Diabetes 2015;6(8):1065–72.
24. Ferrara A. Increasing prevalence of gestational diabetes mellitus: a public health perspective. Diabetes Care 2007;30(Suppl 2):S141–6.
25. Wong LF, Caughey AB, Nakagawa S, et al. Perinatal outcomes among different Asian-American subgroups. Am J Obstet Gynecol 2008;199(4):382.e1-6.
26. Caughey AB, Cheng YW, Stotland NE, et al. Maternal and paternal race/ethnicity are both associated with gestational diabetes. Am J Obstet Gynecol 2010;202(6): 616.e1-5.
27. Powe CE, Allard C, Battista M-C, et al. Heterogeneous Contribution of Insulin Sensitivity and Secretion Defects to Gestational Diabetes Mellitus. Diabetes Care 2016;39(6):1052–5.
28. Kitzmiller JL, Dang-Kilduff L, Taslimi MM. Gestational Diabetes After Delivery: Short-term management and long-term risks. Diabetes Care 2007; 30(Supplement 2):S225–35.
29. Metzger BE, Cho NH, Roston SM, et al. Prepregnancy Weight and Antepartum Insulin Secretion Predict Glucose Tolerance Five Years After Gestational Diabetes Mellitus. Diabetes Care 1993;16(12):1598–605.
30. Bernstein J, Lee-Parritz A, Quinn E, et al. After Gestational Diabetes: Impact of Pregnancy Interval on Recurrence and Type 2 Diabetes. Biores Open Access 2019;8(1):59–64.
31. Song C, Lyu Y, Li C, et al. Long-term risk of diabetes in women at varying durations after gestational diabetes: a systematic review and meta-analysis with more than 2 million women. Obes Rev 2018;19(3):421–9.
32. Poola-Kella S, Steinman RA, Mesmar B, et al. Gestational diabetes mellitus: postpartum risk and follow up. Rev Recent Clin Trials 2018;13(1):5–14.
33. Allalou A, Nalla A, Prentice KJ, et al. A predictive metabolic signature for the transition from gestational diabetes mellitus to type 2 diabetes. Diabetes 2016;65(9): 2529–39.
34. El Ouahabi H, Doubi S, Boujraf S, et al. Gestational diabetes and risk of developing postpartum type 2 diabetes: how to improve follow-up? Int J Prev Med 2019;10:51.
35. Rayanagoudar G, Hashi AA, Zamora J, et al. Quantification of the type 2 diabetes risk in women with gestational diabetes: a systematic review and meta-analysis of 95,750 women. Diabetologia 2016;59(7):1403–11.
36. Köhler M, Ziegler AG, Beyerlein A. Development of a simple tool to predict the risk of postpartum diabetes in women with gestational diabetes mellitus. Acta Diabetol 2016;53(3):433–7.
37. Alberti KGMM, Zimmet P, Shaw J, IDF Epidemiology Task Force Consensus Group. The metabolic syndrome—a new worldwide definition. Lancet 2005; 366(9491):1059–62.
38. Grundy SM, Cleeman JI, Daniels SR, et al. Diagnosis and management of the metabolic syndrome: an American Heart Association/National Heart, Lung, and Blood Institute Scientific Statement. Circulation 2005;112(17):2735–52.
39. Retnakaran R, Qi Y, Connelly PW, et al. Glucose intolerance in pregnancy and postpartum risk of metabolic syndrome in young women. J Clin Endocrinol Metab 2010;95(2):670–7.
40. Retnakaran R, Qi Y, Connelly PW, et al. The graded relationship between glucose tolerance status in pregnancy and postpartum levels of low-density-lipoprotein cholesterol and apolipoprotein B in young women: implications for future cardiovascular risk. J Clin Endocrinol Metab 2010;95(9):4345–53.

41. Lauenborg J, Hansen T, Jensen DM, et al. Increasing incidence of diabetes after gestational diabetes: a long-term follow-up in a Danish population. Diabetes Care 2004;27(5):1194–9.
42. Tobias DK, Hu FB, Forman JP, et al. Increased risk of hypertension after gestational diabetes mellitus: findings from a large prospective cohort study. Diabetes Care 2011;34(7):1582–4.
43. McKenzie-Sampson S, Paradis G, Healy-Profitós J, et al. Gestational diabetes and risk of cardiovascular disease up to 25 years after pregnancy: a retrospective cohort study. Acta Diabetol 2018;55(4):315–22.
44. Ratner RE, Christophi CA, Metzger BE, et al. Prevention of diabetes in women with a history of gestational diabetes: effects of metformin and lifestyle interventions. J Clin Endocrinol Metab 2008;93(12):4774–9.
45. Overview | Diabetes in pregnancy: management from preconception to the postnatal period | Guidance | NICE. Available at: https://www.nice.org.uk/guidance/ng3. Accessed November 25, 2019.
46. Herrick CJ, Keller MR, Trolard AM, et al. Postpartum diabetes screening among low income women with gestational diabetes in Missouri 2010–2015. BMC Public Health 2019;19(1):148.
47. Stasenko M, Cheng YW, McLean T, et al. Postpartum follow-up for women with gestational diabetes mellitus. Am J Perinatol 2010;27(9):737–42.
48. Zapka JG, Puleo E, Taplin SH, et al. Processes of care in cervical and breast cancer screening and follow-up–the importance of communication. Prev Med 2004; 39(1):81–90.
49. Tovar A, Chasan-Taber L, Eggleston E, et al. Postpartum screening for diabetes among women with a history of gestational diabetes mellitus. Prev Chronic Dis 2011;8(6):A124.
50. Ferrara A, Peng T, Kim C. Trends in postpartum diabetes screening and subsequent diabetes and impaired fasting glucose among women with histories of gestational diabetes mellitus: A report from the Translating Research Into Action for Diabetes (TRIAD) Study. Diabetes Care 2009;32(2):269–74.
51. Kim C, McEwen LN, Piette JD, et al. Risk perception for diabetes among women with histories of gestational diabetes mellitus. Diabetes Care 2007;30(9):2281–6.
52. Aziz S, Munim TF, Fatima SS. Post-partum follow-up of women with gestational diabetes mellitus: effectiveness, determinants, and barriers. J Matern Fetal Neonatal Med 2018;31(12):1607–12.
53. McCloskey L, Sherman ML, St John M, et al. Navigating a "perfect storm" on the path to prevention of type 2 diabetes mellitus after gestational diabetes: lessons from patient and provider narratives. Matern Child Health J 2019;23(5):603–12.
54. Castling ZA, Farrell T. An analysis of demographic and pregnancy outcome data to explain non-attendance for postpartum glucose testing in women with gestational diabetes mellitus: Why are patients missing follow-up? Obstet Med 2019; 12(2):85–9.
55. Russell MA, Phipps MG, Olson CL, et al. Rates of postpartum glucose testing after gestational diabetes mellitus. Obstet Gynecol 2006;108(6):1456–62.
56. Bennett WL, Ennen CS, Carrese JA, et al. Barriers to and facilitators of postpartum follow-up care in women with recent gestational diabetes mellitus: a qualitative study. J Womens Health (Larchmt) 2011;20(2):239–45.
57. Koning SH, Lutgers HL, Hoogenberg K, et al. Postpartum glucose follow-up and lifestyle management after gestational diabetes mellitus: general practitioner and patient perspectives. J Diabetes Metab Disord 2016;15:56.

58. Purno NH, Thorpe K, Mukerji G, et al. Effect of postpartum glucose tolerance results on subsequent weight retention in women with recent gestational diabetes: A retrospective cohort study. Diabetes Res Clin Pract 2019;151:169–76.

59. Hunt KJ, Conway DL. Who returns for postpartum glucose screening following gestational diabetes mellitus? Am J Obstet Gynecol 2008;198(4):404.e1-6.

60. Stasenko M, Liddell J, Cheng YW, et al. Patient counseling increases postpartum follow-up in women with gestational diabetes mellitus. Am J Obstet Gynecol 2011;204(6):522.e1-6.

61. Pennington AVR, O'Reilly SL, Young D, et al. Improving follow-up care for women with a history of gestational diabetes: perspectives of GPs and patients. Aust J Prim Health 2017;23(1):66–74.

62. Jeppesen C, Kristensen JK, Ovesen P, et al. The forgotten risk? A systematic review of the effect of reminder systems for postpartum screening for type 2 diabetes in women with previous gestational diabetes. BMC Res Notes 2015;8:373.

63. Clark HD, Graham ID, Karovitch A, et al. Do postal reminders increase postpartum screening of diabetes mellitus in women with gestational diabetes mellitus? A randomized controlled trial. Am J Obstet Gynecol 2009;200(6):634.e1-7.

64. Vesco KK, Dietz PM, Bulkley J, et al. A system-based intervention to improve postpartum diabetes screening among women with gestational diabetes. Am J Obstet Gynecol 2012;207(4):283.e1-6.

65. Su X, Zhang Z, Qu X, et al. Hemoglobin A1c for diagnosis of postpartum abnormal glucose tolerance among women with gestational diabetes mellitus: diagnostic meta-analysis. PLoS One 2014;9(7):e102144.

66. Claesson R, Ignell C, Shaat N, et al. HbA1c as a predictor of diabetes after gestational diabetes mellitus. Prim Care Diabetes 2017;11(1):46–51.

67. Blumer I, Hadar E, Hadden DR, et al. Diabetes and pregnancy: an endocrine society clinical practice guideline. J Clin Endocrinol Metab 2013;98(11):4227–49.

Gestational Weight Gain
Achieving a Healthier Weight Between Pregnancies

Peeraya Sawangkum, MD, Judette M. Louis, MD, MPH*

KEYWORDS

- Excessive gestational weight gain • Obesity • Postpartum weight retention
- Nutrition • Bariatric surgery

KEY POINTS

- Excessive gestational weight gain is correlated with weight retention and subsequent obesity.
- Breastfeeding is associated with less postpartum weight retention.
- Weight optimization in the interconception period is essential in reducing the incidence of long-term obesity.
- Access to family planning services, including effective contraception to aide optimal birth spacing, is an important part of interpregnancy care.
- Multimodal interventions that include diet and exercise and are physician led are associated with less postpartum weight retention.

BACKGROUND

There are 6 classes of body mass index (BMI), defined as weight in kilograms divided by height in meters squared, according to the World Health Organization; these include underweight (BMI <18.5 kg/m^2), normal weight (BMI 18.5–24.9 kg/m^2), overweight (BMI 25.0–29.9 kg/m^2), obesity class I (BMI 30–34.9 kg/m^2), obesity class II (BMI 35.0–39.9 kg/m^2), and obesity class III (BMI >40.0 kg/m^2). It is reported that 31% of reproductive age women are obese (BMI >30.0), and 58% of reproductive age women are at least overweight (BMI >25.0 kg/m^2).[1]

In 2009, the National Academy of Medicine published recommendations for appropriate weight gain in pregnancy.[2] These guidelines harkened a move to individualizing recommendations for gestational weight gain based on a patient's prepregnancy weight. The recommendations recognized different goals for underweight, normal

Department of Obstetrics and Gynecology, University of South Florida, 6th Floor, 2 Tampa General Circle, Tampa, FL 33606, USA
* Corresponding author.
E-mail address: Jlouis1@usf.edu
Twitter: @judettelouis (J.M.L.)

Obstet Gynecol Clin N Am 47 (2020) 397–407
https://doi.org/10.1016/j.ogc.2020.04.003
0889-8545/20/© 2020 Elsevier Inc. All rights reserved.

weight, overweight, and obese patients **(Table 1)**.[2] These same guidelines also detailed trimester-specific weight gain recommendations for each BMI class and provide useful information when counseling patients on appropriate weight gain.[3]

EXCESSIVE GESTATIONAL WEIGHT GAIN

Excessive gestational weight gain is defined as gaining more than the IOM recommended weight during pregnancy. Approximately half of all women exceed the recommended gestational weight gain recommendations.[4] Excessive gestational weight gain has been associated with an increased risk of pregnancy complications, including pregnancy-related hypertension, cesarean delivery regardless of prepregnancy BMI, and large-for-gestational-age infants.[5,6] Beyond the acute risks to the pregnancy there also are future implications. Excessive gestational weight gain is a major risk factor for short-term and long-term postpartum weight retention (PPWR).[7]

Risk factors for excessive gestational weight gain include prepregnancy obesity, low income, and a variety of psychosocial factors, including depression, lack of social support, and stress.[8] A review of 12 published studies examining risk factors for excessive gestational weight gain found the 2 most common factors implicated in excessive gestational weight gain were prepregnancy obesity and poor diet and exercise habits during pregnancy.[8] Low-income women often have poor access to healthy food, are more susceptible to lack of physical activity, and have lower health literacy regarding healthy food choices.[9] All of the challenges interplay and create barriers to optimizing gestational weight gain.

POSTPARTUM WEIGHT RETENTION AND THE CYCLE OF INCREASING BODY MASS INDEX

PPWR is the difference between postpartum weight and prepregnancy weight. After excessive pregnancy weight gain, many women have increased difficulty losing this weight after pregnancy.[4] Although the degree of PPWR is highly variable between women, patients with excess gestational weight gain retain the most weight postpartum.[4,10] Women who are overweight and obese in the preconception period are more likely to experience PPWR, and only 11% of overweight and obese pregnant women return to their preconception weight within 5 years postpartum.[4] A meta-analysis published in 2011 investigated the relationship between gestational weight gain and PPWR; results showed that women with excessive gestational weight gain retained on average an additional 3.06 kg, 3 years postpartum, and 4.72 kg, 15 years postpartum.[11] It is this very PPWR that can lead to a cycle of increasing BMI in

Table 1		
Institute of Medicine recommended gestational weight gain		
Prepregnancy Weight Category	Body Mass Index Range	Recommended Weight Gain (lb)
Underweight	<18.5	28–40
Normal	18.5–24.9	25–35
Overweight	25.0–29.9	15–25
Obese	>30	11–20

Institute of Medicine and National Research Council. 2009. Weight Gain During Pregnancy: Reexamining the Guidelines. https://doi.org/10.17226/12584. *Adapted and reproduced* with permission from the National Academy of Sciences, Courtesy of the National Academies Press, Washington, D.C.

subsequent pregnancies and ultimately long term; women who retain weight in the postpartum period obviously enter a subsequent pregnancy at a higher BMI than in the previous pregnancy, which, in turn, results in greater risk of excessive gestational weight gain and subsequent PPWR. Excessive PPWR during childbearing years is associated with the development of long-term adverse maternal health outcomes, such as cardiovascular diseases, metabolic syndromes, and long-term obesity in later life.[12]

OBESITY AND EXCESSIVE GESTATIONAL WEIGHT GAIN

Obese women are at increased risk of maternal morbidity, cesarean deliveries, failed trial of labor, wound complications, infection, and venous thrombosis.[13] They also have higher rates of miscarriage and stillbirth[14] These adverse outcomes are complicated further by excessive gestational weight gain. Excessive gestational weight gain is associated with hypertensive disorders of pregnancy, including gestational hypertension and preeclampsia.[15,16] Some studies also indicate an association between excessive gestational weight gain and the development of gestational diabetes but other studies have not found that association.[5,17] One study indicated that the timing of the gestational weight gain may have an impact on the outcomes. In a 2012 study, including 7985 nulliparous, low-risk women, early gestational weight gain (that is, weight gain exceeding the IOM recommended weight gain at 15–18 weeks' gestation) was associated with increased odds of developing gestational diabetes compared with nulliparous, low-risk women who did not exhibit early gestational weight gain.[16] Overall, given the varying diagnostic criteria for gestational diabetes, it is difficult to collate the existing studies of excessive gestational weight gain and gestational diabetes. A recent meta-analysis of gestational weight gain and adverse outcomes was unable to comment on gestational diabetes as an outcome.[18]

FUTURE MATERNAL HEALTH

Adverse outcomes in pregnancy have implications for maternal future health. Women with hypertensive disease in pregnancy are twice as likely to develop cardiovascular disease (such as hypertension, myocardial infarction, and congestive heart failure), cerebrovascular events, peripheral arterial disease, and cardiovascular mortality later in life compared with women without hypertensive disease in pregnancy.[19] Similar observations have been made for other adverse pregnancy complications, including gestational diabetes, preterm delivery, fetal growth restriction, and placental abruption.[20,21] The increased risk of cardiovascular disease can be observed as early as 3 years to 5 years after delivery.[22] Given these associations, there has been a focus on using the interpregnancy period to improve maternal health and address modifiable risk factors for cardiovascular disease, such as obesity.[23,24]

TIMING OF INTERVENTIONS

Throughout time, several tools have been studied, with the goal of reducing pregnancy weight gain and PPWR (**Table 2**). There are few longitudinal studies in which there are long-term follow-up and evaluation on maternal weight. This section reviews some interventions and the evidence base for their effectiveness.

Prepregnancy/Interpregnancy

Interventions to prevent long-term pregnancy weight retentions should begin in the prepregnancy period. Prepregnancy counseling is a key tool used to reducing adverse outcomes for women and neonates.[25] The core of preconception counseling involves

Table 2
Tools to limit gestational weight gain and postpartum weight retention

	Prepregnancy	Interpregnancy	Prenatal	Postpartum
Counseling	x	X	X	X
Lifestyle modification	x	X	X	X
Diet and exercise	x	X	X	X
Bariatric surgery	x	X		X
Breastfeeding	x	X		X
Contraception	x	X		X

working with patients to optimize health, address risk factors, and provide education about healthy pregnancy before pregnancy begins. The American College of Obstetricians and Gynecologists recommends the following:

1. Any patient encounter with nonpregnant women or men with reproductive potential is an opportunity to counsel about wellness and healthy eating habits.
2. Patients should be screened regarding diet and vitamin supplements to confirm they are meeting recommended daily allowances.
3. Patients should be encouraged to attain normal BMI before attempting pregnancy.[25]

For overweight and obese women, reducing weight prior to pregnancy can help reduce excessive gestational weight gain as well as decrease the risk of other pregnancy complications.

The US Preventive Services Task Force recommends that all obese adults be referred to multicomponent behavior interventions.[26] Weight management strategies include dietary control, exercise, weight loss medication use, and behavior modification, either alone or in combination.[26–28]

Prenatal Care

Given the role of gestational weight gain in the long-term development of obesity, it is prudent to limit excessive gestational weight gain. Although prenatal providers may be aware of weight gain recommendations and even initiate and document counseling during prenatal visits, the quality and content of such conversations may be limited. Many prenatal care providers consider obesity and excessive gestational weight gain sensitive topics and feel that counseling will not alter women's weight gain trajectory.[25,26] Additional barriers to counseling include time limitations during traditional prenatal care appointments.[27]

One proposed intervention for increasing ease and efficiency of counseling is use of technology to assist providers and patients. Many electronic medical record systems incorporate tools, alerts, and patient education handouts; these can be used to counsel patients on total weight gain recommendations, weekly weight gain goals, templates for prenatal care provider counseling statements, and patient handouts.[26]

Under the standard models of care, prenatal care alone is insufficient to prevent excessive gestational weight gain.[29] Group prenatal care has been proposed as an alternative. In that model of care, patients receive care in a group setting and have reported higher rates of empowerment, self empowerment and self efficacy. Certain high-risk groups, such as adolescents blacks, and Hispanic gravidas, have been shown to benefit from group prenatal care in regard to improved rates of depression symptoms, chronic disease management, and breastfeeding.[30] Those benefits have not extended, however, to gestational weight gain.[31] Further research is needed to determine the relationship between group prenatal care, obesity, and excessive gestational weight gain.

Postpartum Care

After childbirth, most patients in the United States are not scheduled for follow-up care for up to 6 weeks postpartum; furthermore, as many as 40% of all women do not ever attend a postpartum visit, especially those with limited resources.[3,32,33]

Strategies that can be utilized to increase compliance with postpartum follow-up include counseling patients on the importance of postpartum care during preconception counseling and prenatal visits, postpartum discharge planners, scheduling postpartum appointments at prenatal visits (if a patient's delivery date is predetermined, as is the case for scheduled inductions of labor or cesarean delivery), scheduling postpartum appointments prior to hospital discharge, and utilizing technology for appointment reminders.[34]

Chronic health conditions, including obesity, should be addressed at the postpartum visit. This visit should include coordination of care to primary care providers (if necessary) or other subspecialists, such as cardiologists, nutritionist, bariatric care providers, and endocrinologists, to promote health optimization in the postpartum state and/or prior to the next pregnancy.[35]

INTERVENTIONS FOR OBESITY
Lifestyle Interventions

With regard to health, lifestyle refers to dietary habits; physical activity habits; the social use of substances, such as alcohol and tobacco; and exposure to other risky behaviors. Lifestyle interventions are effective in achieving 5% to 10% weight loss and improving outcomes in obesity-related diseases.[36] Lifestyle interventions that target pregnancy-related weight recently have been focused on reducing gestational weight gain. One example, Lifestyle Interventions for Expectant Moms, is a consortium of 7 independent but collaborative clinical trials that sought to evaluate the efficacy of varied lifestyle intervention programs designed to decrease excessive gestational weight gain compared with standard care. The primary hypothesis was that lifestyle interventions targeting diet, physical activity, and behavioral strategies in women with overweight and obesity would reduce excess gestational weight gain as defined by IOM recommendations. The interventions varied and included meal replacements, modified Diabetes Prevention Program intervention, the Dietary Approaches to Stop Hypertension (DASH) diet, smartphone-based intervention, and parent educator intervention.[37] Although the intervention group was effective in reducing gestational weight gain, the effect size was modest when compared to routine care (9.7 kg $\pm$ 5.4 vs.8.1 kg $\pm$ 5.2 kg; $P<.001$), respectively.[37]

Exercise

Regular physical exercise was more likely to help prevent excessive gestational weight gain and postpartum retention of weight after birth than traditional medical care that did not include exercise.[38] In a systematic review, 11 published randomized clinical trials contained useable information on PPWR but were scored low to moderate quality due to inconsistencies in intervention and outcomes measures. Exercise only compared with no exercise was associated with less postpartum retention but the effect size is modest for both gestational weight gain and PPWR (-0.85 kg; 95% CI, -1.46 kg to -0.25 kg) The most benefit of exercise as an intervention is demonstrated among women who exercise 3 times per week or more.[39] In pregnancies affected by gestational diabetes, it has been shown that the addition of physical exertion to dietary modification helps lower blood glucose and reduce insulin requirement.[40]

A significant limitation exists currently in the literature because most studies focused on women without underlying medical concerns or pregnancy complications. More studies urgently are needed to evaluate the role of exercise in women with underlying medical comorbidities or pregnancy complications. These populations are particularly in need of interventions on the interpregnancy and postpartum periods to optimize their health. Nevertheless, it is imperative that health care providers emphasize the importance of appropriate physical activity in pregnancy and subsequent transition of pregnancy habits to lifelong lifestyle modification.[34]

Implementation of Weight Loss Programs

The complexity of weight loss means that there is not 1 clear solution for effectiveness. Multicomponent approaches, including a balanced diet with low glycemic load and light to moderate intensity physical activity, 30 minutes to 60 minutes per day for 3 days to 5 days per week, seem more effective than using 1 component.[41] A review of the existing studies of postpartum interventions indicates that health professional–delivered interventions were associated with greater weight loss than those delivered by nonhealth professionals (mean difference, 95% CI, -3.22 kg [-4.83 to -1.61] vs -0.99 kg [-1.53 to -0.45]; $P = .01$, respectively). Diet and physical activity combined were associated with greater weight loss compared with physical activity–only interventions (95% CI, -3.15 kg [-4.34 to -1.96] vs -0.78 kg [-1.73 to 0.16]; $P = .009$, respectively).[42] Interventions also were more likely to be successful if objective goals were used, such as the use of heart rate monitors or pedometer and exercise combined with intensive dietary intervention. There is benefit from overall lifestyle interventions on weight loss in postpartum women, and exercise plus intensive diet and objective targets are the most effective intervention strategies. These components should be considered when formulating an intervention plan with patients.[42]

Bariatric Surgery

Bariatric surgery presents an opportunity for effective weight loss among obese women.[43] Pregnant women with a pregnancy within less than 12 months of bariatric surgery compared with women who have had surgery greater than 12 months prior to pregnancy have less gestational weight gain (4.9 kg vs 10.9 kg; $P = .01$, respectively) and PPWR (-1.3 kg vs 8.3 kg; $P = .02$, respectively).[44] The impacts of pregnancy on long-term weight loss are less clear and challenged by differences in bariatric surgery technique and duration of follow-up.[45,46] One study of 591 women who had undergone a laparoscopic gastric band or a Roux-en-Y procedure found that women who had a pregnancy compared with women who did not have a pregnancy had a slower rate of weight loss. At the 5-year follow-up period, however, both groups had similar rates of excess weight loss (47.7% $\pm$ 27.7% vs 49.9% $\pm$ 28.9%; $P = .644$, respectively).

Breastfeeding

The 2016 Centers for Disease Control and Prevention data indicate a majority of women (83%) initiate breastfeeding. At 6 months and 1 year postpartum, however, breastfeeding rates decline substantially to 57% and 36%, respectively.[47] In addition to providing benefits to infant health and improving maternal-infant bonding, breastfeeding has been associated with a return to normal weight in the postpartum period.

From 0 to 6 months postpartum, breastfeeding women expend an extra 300 kcal per day compared with non-breastfeeding women; from 7 months to 12 months postpartum, breastfeeding women expend an extra 400 kcal per day compared with non-breastfeeding women.[48] Although women who breastfeed are more likely to return to a normal weight, it has been difficult to prove causation. Increased caloric expenditure and decreased cost (as women do not have to pay for breastmilk) can greatly facilitate postpartum weight loss by potentially allowing patients to spend money on healthy foods as opposed to infant formula.

Motivational Interviewing

Motivational interviewing, a technique recommended by American College of Obstetricians and Gynecologists (ACOG), has been demonstrated to help limit gestational weight gain. It is "a directive, patient-centered counseling style for eliciting behavior change by helping patients explore and resolve ambivalence."[37] It relies heavily on identifying the stages of readiness for change and helping patients move through the stages of change to achieve a desired behavior using techniques to help patients develop new thought patterns (**Box 1**). Core techniques include the following:

1. Expressing empathy and avoiding arguments
2. Developing discrepancies (ie, helping patients understand the differences between their behavior and their goals)
3. Rolling with resistance and providing personalized feedback
4. Supporting self-efficacy and eliciting self-motivation[49]

Patient Navigation

Patient navigation is the use of trained personnel to promote health care access and utilization.[50] The use of patient navigation in the postpartum period has been associated with improvements in depression screening, contraception uptake, and vaccination.[51] Given the unique stressors of the postpartum period and the success of patient navigation, it has been suggested as a mechanism for improving postpartum weight loss. This failed to be the case in a prospective study of women who participated in a postpartum patient navigation program designed to improve uptake of postpartum care. Among the 152 primarily low-income and racial/ethnic minority women in the patient navigation program and 159 historical controls, there was no difference at 4 weeks to 12 weeks postpartum, mean PPWR (4.0 kg $\pm$ 6.7 kg vs 2.7 kg $\pm$ 6.3 kg; $P = .06$, respectively) and PPWR greater than 5 kg (61/144 [42%] vs 50/145 [34%]; $P = .15$, respectively). Up to 12 months postpartum, the mean PPWR (4.5 kg $\pm$ 7.1 kg vs 5.0 kg $\pm$ 7.5 kg; $P = .59$, respectively) and PPWR greater than 5 kg (22/

Box 1
Stages of readiness for change

- Precontemplation—the patient does not believe a problem exists.
- Contemplation—the patient recognizes a problem exists and is considering treatment or behavior change.
- Action—the patient begins treatment or behavior change.
- Maintenance—the patient incorporates new behavior into daily life.
- Relapse—the patient returns to the undesired behavior.

50 [44%] vs 30/57 [53%]; $P = .55$, respectively) did not differ between groups. The findings indicate that providing social support is not enough to effect weight change in the postpartum period.[52]

Birth Spacing

Approximately 45% of all pregnancies in the United States are unintended.[53] Given that prepregnancy obesity is one of the top risk factors for excessive gestational weight gain, a logical point of impact in addressing this public health problem is preconception counseling and health optimization prior to pregnancy. Necessary to this is access to contraception and abortion services, especially within the interpregnancy period.[54] In January 2019, the ACOG released an Obstetric Care Consensus, which made recommendations for interpregnancy care for women who desired future pregnancies.[35] Recommendations within this document include the following:

1. Women should be advised to avoid interpregnancy intervals shorter than 6 months.
2. Women should be counseled about the risks and benefits of repeat pregnancy sooner than 18 months.
3. Family planning counseling should begin during prenatal care with a conversation about the women's interest in future childbearing.[35]

Contraception counseling should begin as soon as possible during prenatal care and continue throughout the postpartum period to allow patients to make an autonomous, informed decision and achieve health optimization prior to the subsequent pregnancy.[35] Women also should have access to all contraceptive methods in the immediate postpartum period; long-acting reversible contraceptives in particular may be helpful in reducing unplanned pregnancy and optimizing birth spacing.[55,56]

SUMMARY

Excessive gestational weight gain is associated with an increased risk of PPWR and long-term obesity. Although preconception and prenatal counseling are essential for helping women achieving healthier weight in pregnancy, postpartum and interpregnancy care remains important as well. Lifestyle interventions have been successful in reducing gestational weight gain. Postpartum interventions that can help women achieve a healthier weight include contraception counseling and access, encouragement of breastfeeding, and referral to nutrition and dietary services. Beyond the examination room, obstetricians and gynecologists can work as advocates for patient health and organize for policies that promote broader health insurance coverage beyond pregnancy and expand access to family planning services to allow for patient autonomy and healthier pregnancy spacing.

DISCLOSURE

The authors have nothing to disclose.

REFERENCES

1. ACOG committee opinion no. 763: ethical considerations for the care of patients with obesity. Obstet Gynecol 2019;133(1):e90–6.
2. Institute of Medicine, National Research Council Committee to Reexamine IOMPWG. The National Academies Collection: Reports funded by National Institutes of Health. In: Rasmussen KM, Yaktine AL, editors. Weight gain during

pregnancy: reexamining the guidelines. Washington (DC): National Academies Press (US) National Academy of Sciences.; 2009.

3. ACOG Committee opinion no. 548: weight gain during pregnancy. Obstet Gynecol 2013;121(1):210–2.

4. Gilmore LA, Klempel-Donchenko M, Redman LM. Pregnancy as a window to future health: Excessive gestational weight gain and obesity. Semin Perinatol 2015;39(4):296–303.

5. McDowell M, Cain MA, Brumley J. Excessive gestational weight gain. J Midwifery Womens Health 2019;64(1):46–54.

6. Dude AM, Grobman W, Haas D, et al. Gestational weight gain and pregnancy outcomes among nulliparous women. Am J Perinatol 2019. [Epub ahead of print].

7. Mamun AA, Kinarivala M, O'Callaghan MJ, et al. Associations of excess weight gain during pregnancy with long-term maternal overweight and obesity: evidence from 21 y postpartum follow-up. Am J Clin Nutr 2010;91(5):1336–41.

8. Samura T, Steer J, Michelis LD, et al. Factors Associated With Excessive Gestational Weight Gain: Review of Current Literature. Glob Adv Health Med 2016;5(1): 87–93.

9. Kwarteng JL, Schulz AJ, Mentz GB, et al. Independent Effects of Neighborhood Poverty and Psychosocial Stress on Obesity Over Time. J Urban Health 2017; 94(6):791–802.

10. Chagas DCD, Silva A, Ribeiro CCC, et al. [Effects of gestational weight gain and breastfeeding on postpartum weight retention among women in the BRISA cohort]. Cad Saude Publica 2017;33(5):e00007916.

11. Nehring I, Schmoll S, Beyerlein A, et al. Gestational weight gain and long-term postpartum weight retention: a meta-analysis. Am J Clin Nutr 2011;94(5): 1225–31.

12. Linne Y, Neovius M. Identification of women at risk of adverse weight development following pregnancy. Int J Obes (Lond) 2006;30(8):1234–9.

13. Dolin CD, Kominiarek MA. Pregnancy in Women with Obesity. Obstet Gynecol Clin North Am 2018;45(2):217–32.

14. Salihu HM, Dunlop AL, Hedayatzadeh M, et al. Extreme obesity and risk of stillbirth among black and white gravidas. Obstet Gynecol 2007;110(3):552–7.

15. Premru-Srsen T, Kocic Z, Fabjan Vodusek V, et al. Total gestational weight gain and the risk of preeclampsia by pre-pregnancy body mass index categories: a population-based cohort study from 2013 to 2017. J Perinat Med 2019;47(6): 585–91.

16. Santos S, Voerman E, Amiano P, et al. Impact of maternal body mass index and gestational weight gain on pregnancy complications: an individual participant data meta-analysis of European, North American and Australian cohorts. BJOG 2019;126(8):984–95.

17. Jin C, Lin L, Han N, et al. Excessive gestational weight gain and the risk of gestational diabetes: Comparison of Intergrowth-21st standards, IOM recommendations and a local reference. Diabetes Res Clin Pract 2019;158:107912.

18. Goldstein RF, Abell SK, Ranasinha S, et al. Association of Gestational Weight Gain With Maternal and Infant Outcomes: A Systematic Review and Meta-analysis. JAMA 2017;317(21):2207–25.

19. Behrens I, Basit S, Melbye M, et al. Risk of post-pregnancy hypertension in women with a history of hypertensive disorders of pregnancy: nationwide cohort study. BMJ 2017;358:j3078.

20. Smith GN, Louis JM, Saade GR. Pregnancy and the Postpartum Period as an Opportunity for Cardiovascular Risk Identification and Management. Obstet Gynecol 2019;134(4):851–62.
21. Hauspurg A, Ying W, Hubel CA, et al. Adverse pregnancy outcomes and future maternal cardiovascular disease. Clin Cardiol 2018;41(2):239–46.
22. Cain MA, Salemi JL, Tanner JP, et al. Pregnancy as a window to future health: maternal placental syndromes and short-term cardiovascular outcomes. Am J Obstet Gynecol 2016;215(4):484.e1-4.
23. Gladstone RA, Pudwell J, Nerenberg KA, et al. Cardiovascular Risk Assessment and Follow-Up of Women After Hypertensive Disorders of Pregnancy:A Prospective Cohort Study. J Obstet Gynaecol Can 2019;41(8):1157–67.e1.
24. Cusimano MC, Pudwell J, Roddy M, et al. The maternal health clinic: an initiative for cardiovascular risk identification in women with pregnancy-related complications. Am J Obstet Gynecol 2014;210(5):438.e1-9.
25. ACOG Committee Opinion No. 762: Prepregnancy Counseling. Obstet Gynecol 2019;133(1):e78–89.
26. AHRQ. Screening for and Management of Obesity. 2015. Available at: https://www.ahrq.gov/ncepcr/tools/healthier-pregnancy/fact-sheets/obesity.html. Accessed December 1, 2019.
27. LeBlanc ES, Patnode CD, Webber EM, et al. Behavioral and Pharmacotherapy Weight Loss Interventions to Prevent Obesity-Related Morbidity and Mortality in Adults: Updated Evidence Report and Systematic Review for the US Preventive Services Task Force. JAMA 2018;320(11):1172–91.
28. Tronieri JS, Wadden TA, Chao AM, et al. Primary Care Interventions for Obesity: Review of the Evidence. Curr Obes Rep 2019;8(2):128–36.
29. Yeo S, Crandell JL, Jones-Vessey K. Adequacy of Prenatal Care and Gestational Weight Gain. J Womens Health (Larchmt) 2016;25(2):117–23.
30. Byerley BM, Haas DM. A systematic overview of the literature regarding group prenatal care for high-risk pregnant women. BMC Pregnancy Childbirth 2017; 17(1):329.
31. Brumley J, Cain MA, Stern M, et al. Gestational Weight Gain and Breastfeeding Outcomes in Group Prenatal Care. J Midwifery Womens Health 2016;61(5): 557–62.
32. Tully KP, Stuebe AM, Verbiest SB. The fourth trimester: a critical transition period with unmet maternal health needs. Am J Obstet Gynecol 2017;217(1):37–41.
33. Bennett WL, Chang HY, Levine DM, et al. Utilization of primary and obstetric care after medically complicated pregnancies: an analysis of medical claims data. J Gen Intern Med 2014;29(4):636–45.
34. Nascimento SL, Surita FG, Cecatti JG. Physical exercise during pregnancy: a systematic review. Curr Opin Obstet Gynecol 2012;24(6):387–94.
35. Louis JM, Bryant A, Ramos D, et al. Interpregnancy Care. Am J Obstet Gynecol 2019;220(1):B2–18.
36. Marek RJ, Coulon SM, Brown JD, et al. Characteristics of Weight Loss Trajectories in a Comprehensive Lifestyle Intervention. Obesity (Silver Spring) 2017; 25(12):2062–7.
37. Peaceman AM, Clifton RG, Phelan S, et al. Lifestyle Interventions Limit Gestational Weight Gain in Women with Overweight or Obesity: LIFE-Moms Prospective Meta-Analysis. Obesity (Silver Spring) 2018;26(9):1396–404.
38. Ruchat S-M, Mottola MF, Skow RJ, et al. Effectiveness of exercise interventions in the prevention of excessive gestational weight gain and postpartum weight

retention: a systematic review and meta-analysis. Br J Sports Med 2018;52(21): 1347–56.

39. Wang J, Wen D, Liu X, et al. Impact of exercise on maternal gestational weight gain: An updated meta-analysis of randomized controlled trials. Medicine (Baltimore) 2019;98(27):e16199.

40. Nartea R, Mitoiu BI, Nica AS. Correlation between Pregnancy Related Weight Gain, Postpartum Weight loss and Obesity: a Prospective Study. J Med Life 2019;12(2):178–83.

41. Farpour-Lambert NJ, Ells LJ, Martinez de Tejada B, et al. Obesity and Weight Gain in Pregnancy and Postpartum: an Evidence Review of Lifestyle Interventions to Inform Maternal and Child Health Policies. Front Endocrinol 2018;9:546.

42. Lim S, Liang X, Hill B, et al. A systematic review and meta-analysis of intervention characteristics in postpartum weight management using the TIDieR framework: A summary of evidence to inform implementation. Obes Rev 2019;20(7):1045–56.

43. Maciejewski ML, Arterburn DE, Van Scoyoc L, et al. Bariatric Surgery and Long-term Durability of Weight Loss. JAMA Surg 2016;151(11):1046–55.

44. Dolin CD, Chervenak J, Pivo S, et al. Association between time interval from bariatric surgery to pregnancy and maternal weight outcomes. J Matern Fetal Neonatal Med 2019;1–7.

45. Rottenstreich A, Shufanieh J, Kleinstern G, et al. The long-term effect of pregnancy on weight loss after sleeve gastrectomy. Surg Obes Relat Dis 2018; 14(10):1594–9.

46. Froylich D, Corcelles R, Daigle CR, et al. The effect of pregnancy before and/or after bariatric surgery on weight loss. Surg Obes Relat Dis 2016;12(3):596–9.

47. CDC. Breastfeeding among U.S. children born 2009–2016, CDC National Immunization Survey. Available at: https://www.cdc.gov/breastfeeding/data/nis_data/results.html. Accessed December 1, 2019.

48. Kominiarek MA, Rajan P. Nutrition recommendations in pregnancy and lactation. Med Clin North Am 2016;100(6):1199–215.

49. ACOG committee opinion no. 650: physical activity and exercise during pregnancy and the postpartum period. Obstet Gynecol 2015;126(6):e135–42.

50. McKenney KM, Martinez NG, Yee LM. Patient navigation across the spectrum of women's health care in the United States. Am J Obstet Gynecol 2018;218(3): 280–6.

51. Yee LM, Martinez NG, Nguyen AT, et al. Using a patient navigator to improve postpartum care in an urban Women's Health Clinic. Obstet Gynecol 2017; 129(5):925–33.

52. Kominiarek MA, Summerlin S, Martinez NG, et al. Postpartum Patient Navigation and Postpartum Weight Retention. AJP Rep 2019;9(3):e292–7.

53. Finer LB, Zolna MR. Declines in Unintended Pregnancy in the United States, 2008-2011. N Engl J Med 2016;374(9):843–52.

54. Thiel de Bocanegra H, Chang R, Howell M, et al. Interpregnancy intervals: impact of postpartum contraceptive effectiveness and coverage. Am J Obstet Gynecol 2014;210(4):311.e1-8.

55. Winner B, Peipert JF, Zhao Q, et al. Effectiveness of long-acting reversible contraception. N Engl J Med 2012;366(21):1998–2007.

56. Vricella LK, Gawron LM, Louis JM. Society for Maternal-Fetal Medicine (SMFM) Consult Series #48: Immediate postpartum long-acting reversible contraception for women at high risk for medical complications. Am J Obstet Gynecol 2019; 220(5):B2–12.

Postpartum Depression
Identification and Treatment in the Clinic Setting

Emily B. Kroska, PhD[a], Zachary N. Stowe, MD[b],*

KEYWORDS

- Postpartum depression • Diagnosis • Prevalence • Antidepressants
- Psychotherapy

KEY POINTS

- Postpartum depression (PPD) is a common disorder that if left untreated may have adverse consequences for women, children, and families.
- A variety of risk factors have been reliably characterized, enabling clinicians to identify women at risk and develop treatment plans for prevention and intervention.
- Use of a screening tool, such as the Edinburgh Postnatal Depression Scale (10-item, self-rated), will improve early identification in the primary care setting.
- Antidepressants and psychotherapies are effective in the treatment of PPD.
- The selective serotonin reuptake inhibitors have a large database for use during pregnancy and breast-feeding.

INTRODUCTION

Postpartum depression (PPD) is broadly defined as an episode of major depression occurring during the perinatal period. PPD affects about 10% to 15% of women in developed countries following childbirth. PPD is the leading cause of nonobstetric hospitalization among childbearing women in the United States.[1] PPD confers a substantial risk to the mother, family, and offspring across several domains. As such, recent initiatives to increase screening and preventive care have been released by the US Preventive Services Task Force.[2,3] The current review addresses the *diagnosis, prevalence, predictors, consequences,* and *treatment* of PPD.

Diagnosis

PPD is not defined as a unique diagnostic code by the *Diagnostic and Statistical Manual (DSM-5).*[4] Instead, a diagnosis of major depressive disorder is given with

[a] Department of Psychological and Brain Sciences, University of Iowa, W311 Seashore Hall, Iowa City, IA 52242, USA; [b] Department of Psychiatry, University of Wisconsin-Madison, 6001 Research Park Boulevard, Madison, WI 53719, USA
* Corresponding author. 6001 Research Park Drive, Madison, WI 63719.
E-mail address: zstowe@wisc.edu

Obstet Gynecol Clin N Am 47 (2020) 409–419
https://doi.org/10.1016/j.ogc.2020.05.001
0889-8545/20/© 2020 Elsevier Inc. All rights reserved.

obgyn.theclinics.com

the specifier "with peripartum onset," which indicates that onset of symptoms is during pregnancy or in the first 4 weeks after delivery.[4] Criteria include 5 of 9 symptoms for most of 2 weeks, clinical impairment, and elimination of alternative causes. In research contexts, the postpartum period is less rigidly defined, with the World Health Organization classifying PPD as occurring during pregnancy or within the 12 months following delivery.

It is clinically important to distinguish from PPD the postpartum blues, which include mood symptoms (eg, tearfulness, lability) in the first 4 to 10 days following delivery. Postpartum blues are considered mild in severity and limited in duration, and most importantly, do not impair functioning.[5] Estimates indicate that most women experience postpartum blues symptoms following childbirth. Furthermore, PPD is also distinct from postpartum psychosis, characterized by severe mood disturbances and psychotic symptoms, and often requiring inpatient hospitalization.[6] Symptoms of anxiety are frequently comorbid with PPD, with some studies suggesting that nearly half of symptoms in late pregnancy and 40% of symptoms in the postpartum were related to anxiety (as measured by the Edinburgh Postnatal Depression Scale [EPDS]).[7] Also observed in this study were elevated obsessive-compulsive symptoms in the perinatal and postpartum assessments as compared with nonpregnant women.[7] Miller and O'Hara[8] found that about 30% of women reported clinically significant obsessive-compulsive symptoms at 2 –weeks' postpartum, and 11% at 12 –weeks' postpartum. Furthermore, intrusive thoughts and compulsive behaviors were associated with worsened depressive symptoms at both 2 and 12 weeks' postpartum.[8]

Prevalence

Given variability in the time course of measurement, assessment methodology, and study sample, prevalence estimates for PPD vary substantially. Frequently, studies use self-report screening instruments to estimate prevalence, which creates substantial variability in estimates across studies and samples. Estimates of prevalence are also impacted by the time interval specified by the investigators as to what constitutes or defines the postpartum period.

A seminal metaanalysis published in 1996 identified a prevalence of 13%[9]; this was followed by a meta-analysis that only included studies that used interview assessments, rather than self-report measures, finding a prevalence of minor or major depression of 19.2% (7.1% for major depression) in the 3 months following delivery.[10] One metaanalysis specifically examined prevalence of PPD symptoms among mothers who were healthy before pregnancy, finding a prevalence of 17%.[11] A recent metaanalysis comparing prevalence across nations found substantial variability among a global pooled prevalence of 17.7%.[12] Importantly, 73% of the variability in prevalence was accounted for by economic and health variability, suggesting the importance of socioeconomic and health disparities in determining risk for PPD.[12]

A question of particular interest that has continued to generate investigation has been whether the prevalence of depression in the postpartum period is elevated relative to the risk for non-postpartum women in the childbearing years. Methods undertaken to study this phenomenon have included pairing pregnant women and closely matched nonpregnant acquaintances through pregnancy and postpartum, finding that risk for depression diagnosis was not elevated among the pregnant women, but higher depressive symptoms were observed late in pregnancy and in the early postpartum.[13] A large population-based study in Sweden calculated relative risk of depression following childbirth as compared with a computer-generated random date unrelated to childbirth, finding that depression was no more likely to occur following childbirth.[14] In contrast, there have been several longitudinal studies indicating that the postpartum period is a time of elevated risk for both depression[15–17] and psychiatric hospital admission.[18] One study examined both trait (susceptibility to develop depression) and state (episodic depressive symptoms) depression across 10 years, finding that when controlling for trait depression, the risk for depression in the postpartum period is elevated, with the highest risk in the first months postpartum.[19] Finally, heritability research has indicated that one-third of the genetic variability in PPD was unique, unshared with nonperinatal depression.[20] Future research should continue to examine relative risk for depression postpartum and account for variables that may compound risk, including perinatal complications.

Predictors of Risk for Postpartum Depression

Substantial research has focused on identification of factors that increase individual risk for development of PPD. A limitation of much of this research is that factors are not often considered in conjunction given small sample sizes within particular categories of risk, limiting statistical power. A recent population-based study addressed such limitations by comparing mothers with and without a history of depression, and as such, identified risk factors within this context.[21] This study identified that a history of depression increased risk for PPD 20-fold.[21] When accounting for history of depression, maternal age conferred increased risk for PPD, both for adolescents with no history of depression and for women 35 years of age and older with a history of depression.[21] Furthermore, a recent metaanalysis indicated an increase in risk for PPD among women with gestational diabetes.[22] Silverman and colleagues[21] found that among those with a history of depression, the risk for PPD increased 1.5-fold. Emotional symptoms in the early postpartum period, such as postpartum blues,[23] as well as high negative affect and low positive affect,[24] predict PPD symptoms longitudinally. **Box 1** summarizes the replicated predictors identified through metaanalysis.

Screening

The US Preventive Services Task Force recommended screening of pregnant and postpartum women to encourage early identification of symptoms, appropriate referral, and

---

Box 1
Risk factors for postpartum depression

History of depression[21,68,69]

Higher maternal age[21]

Shorter gestational age[21]

Gestational diabetes[21,22]

Depression or anxiety symptoms during pregnancy[9,68]

Postpartum blues symptoms[69]

Stressful life events[9,68,69]

Poor quality of marital relationship[9,69]

Poor social support[9,68,69]

Low socioeconomic status[9,12,69]

Low self-esteem[69]

Difficult infant temperament[69]

Unplanned or unwanted pregnancy[69]

treatment.[25] The American College of Obstetricians and Gynecologists recommends use of the EPDS[26] for screening. The scale considers both depressive and anxiety symptoms and measures mood-related symptoms rather than somatic symptoms that may be associated with pregnancy and delivery (eg, lack of sleep, fatigue). Elevated scores ($\geq$10) indicate *possible* PPD and warrant further evaluation. A large study in Ireland found when using a score of greater than 12 on the EPDS, 15.8% of women demonstrated *probable* depression, with higher symptoms later in pregnancy.[27] The final item assesses suicidal ideation and should be given consideration independent of the total score. Suicide contributes significantly to postpartum maternal mortality. Consistent screening for depression during the prenatal and the early postpartum period and with follow-up for women who screen positive could substantially reduce maternal mortality related to suicide. Other scales commonly used for screening include the Patient Health Questionnaire-9[28] and the Beck Depression Inventory.[29]

Another widely used method includes screening for dysphoric mood or anhedonia, and if positive, administration of a depression questionnaire. The US Agency for Healthcare Research and Quality and the United Kingdom's National Institute for Health and Care Excellence both recommend serial testing methodology. The use of this method has proved both sensitive and specific.

Screening with self-report questionnaires should be followed with formal diagnostic assessment and intervention. Evaluation should include assessment of symptoms, duration of symptoms, and clinical impairment. Alternative causes should be ruled out via both clinical interview and laboratory measures (eg, thyroid levels). Symptoms of mania and psychosis should be thoroughly evaluated in order to rule out postpartum psychosis and bipolar disorder. A complete personal and family history should be ascertained. Suicidal ideation, intent, means, and plan should be evaluated, as well as personal and family history of suicidality. Identification of imminent risk requires immediate psychiatric attention, which likely includes hospitalization and subsequent outpatient treatment. Finally, comorbid symptoms, including anxiety, obsessive-compulsive, panic, and substance use symptoms, should be assessed. Appropriate follow-up should be scheduled to monitor symptoms and treatment response.

Consequences

PPD is known to have a broad array of adverse effects on the mother, infant, and family. Although depression is associated with substantial disease burden and disability, PPD may be particularly consequential given the additional demands of child care. Studies indicate that PPD symptoms were the strongest predictor of poorer maternal responsiveness to the infant when including comorbid obsessive-compulsive symptoms and baseline depressive symptoms in the model.[8] Other studies have linked maternal PPD to insecure attachment and poor interaction between mother and child.[30] Poor interactions can impact long-term emotion regulation and distress tolerance, and several studies have conceptualized these abilities as ego-resilience.[31] Children of mothers with PPD had lower cognitive performance at 18 months, and boys were most adversely affected.[32] Child cognitive,[33] social,[31] and behavioral[33,34] functioning also has been shown to be adversely impacted by maternal PPD.

Beyond the impact on the child, PPD is associated with increased risk for psychiatric hospitalization.[18,35] Furthermore, PPD increases risk for maternal suicide if left undiagnosed, or if diagnosed but without follow-up and treatment.[36,37] Among parenting behaviors, PPD has been shown to impact breast-feeding, sleep, health care utilization, and infant vaccinations.[38] PPD also affects the partner of the mother, with increased paternal depression and parenting stress.[39] PPD is also associated with social isolation and marital discord.[40] As such, PPD has a significant impact on the mother but also on family dynamics, which can have long-term consequences.

Treatment

A review of the literature suggested that education about PPD can encourage help-seeking behavior and promote early recognition of symptoms.[41] Several treatments have been identified through randomized trials as effective for reducing PPD symptoms, including both psychotherapy and medications (**Table 1**).

Table 1 Treatment of postpartum depression	
Psychotherapy	**Medication**
Cognitive-behavioral therapy[a]	Sertraline[a]
Interpersonal psychotherapy[a]	Fluoxetine[a]
Listening visits[a]	Paroxetine[a]
Supportive counseling	Escitalopram
	Fluvoxamine
	Venlafaxine
	Nortriptyline
	Bupropion
	Nefazodone
	Brexanolone[a]

[a] Indicates support by at least 1 randomized controlled trial.

Psychotherapy

Cognitive behavioral therapy (CBT) has demonstrated the most short- and long-term effectiveness when compared with treatment-as-usual interventions in reducing PPD symptoms in a recent metaanalysis.[42] CBT approaches may include strategies to address dysfunctional patterns of thoughts or promote behavioral engagement. Mindfulness- or acceptance-based CBT approaches may also emphasize changing the way one relates or responds to thoughts or emotions, rather than trying to alter the experience itself.[43]

Interpersonal psychotherapy (IPT) has garnered strong evidence of effectiveness in treating PPD in both individual and group formats.[44,45] IPT is a time-limited approach that contextualizes depression within the woman's relationships, aiming to reduce symptoms, expand interpersonal functioning, and increase social support. One meta-analysis found that when compared with control conditions, IPT had greater effect sizes than CBT.[46]

Other studies investigating supportive counseling approaches have found reductions in PPD.[47] Also based in a client-centered approach are listening visits, an intervention developed in the United Kingdom to be delivered by home visiting nurses.[48] The listening visits intervention has demonstrated effectiveness in treating depression in the United Kingdom, Sweden, and United States.[48–50] It is feasible that these listening interventions could be further facilitated through telemedicine or other media, if available.

Medication

Typically, the first-line medication treatments for PPD are selective serotonin reuptake inhibitors (SSRI),[51] which carry low toxicity risk with regard to potential overdose and are less commonly associated with severe side effects. The SSRIs with the most randomized controlled trials to treat PPD are sertraline[52–54] and fluoxetine.[55] Fluoxetine was superior to placebo and comparable to psychotherapy.[55] Also identified as appropriate for PPD are paroxetine,[56,57] fluvoxamine,[58] and escitalopram.[59] A serotonin-norepinephrine reuptake inhibitor, venlafaxine,[60] is supported for treatment of PPD. As a class, antidepressants, particularly the SSRIs, have the largest database in breast-feeding and appear largely devoid of adverse effects. The most detailed data on nursing infant exposure through human breast milk rest with sertraline.[61]

Tricyclic antidepressants are not a first-line treatment and are considered high risk for potential overdose. In this class, nortriptyline has demonstrated preliminary indications of treating PPD.[51] Other medications that have been used in treating PPD include buproprion[62] and nefazodone.[63] Nortriptyline, bupropion, and nefazodone have not been examined in randomized trials, and thus, conclusions regarding effectiveness cannot be drawn.

It is important to educate patients that all aforementioned medication treatments for PPD often require several adherent weeks to be beneficial. As such, it is important to

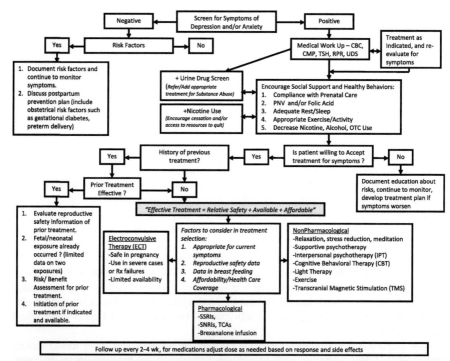

Fig. 1. Guidelines for identification and treatment planning for women during the perinatal period, modified from www.angelsguidelines.com. CBC, complete blood count; CMP, comprehensive metabolic panel; OTC, over the counter; Rx, prescription; TCAs, tricyclic antidepressants; TSH, thyroid stimulating hormone; PNV, prenatal vitamin; RPR, rapid plasma regain; UDS, urine drug screen; SSRI, selective serotonin re-uptake inhibitors; SNRI, serotonin / norepinephrine re-uptake inhibitors. (*Adapted from* The Antenatal and Neonatal Guidelines, Education and Learning System (ANGELS). Treatment of depression in pregnancy and postpartum period. ANGELS was established by two major state agencies, the University of Arkansas College of Medicine and the Arkansas Department of Human. www.angelsguidelines.com.)

have follow-up to determine effectiveness of the treatment regimen in improving symptoms as the mother is attempting to navigate the many challenges that might present in the first months following childbirth. This follow-up is especially important for the mother who has given birth to a preterm infant, the mother who has given birth to an infant with a birth defect, or the mother who has given birth to a child with physical or emotional needs. A new treatment offering a solution to this limitation of other treatments is allopregnanolone (Brexanolone), which modulates GABA type A receptors. Recent trials indicated reductions in depressive symptoms in as early as 60 hours.[64,65] The major limitation of this medication is the considerable time and monitoring required for administration (ie, 60 hours of intravenous infusion). However, this drug is the first drug approved by the Food and Drug Administration (March 2019) specifically for treatment of PPD.

It is important for clinicians to consider treatment planning for preventing PPD in high-risk populations. A recent review[66] provided a summary of the available literature, including a randomized trial of sertraline that demonstrated dramatic efficacy in the prevention of PPD.[67] Identification of at-risk populations and incorporation of additional risk factors over the course of pregnancy and childbirth can better determine those women who are candidates for preventative treatment.

Several information sites are available to support clinicians in the identification and treatment planning for women during the perinatal period, such as www. angelsguidelines.com. **Fig. 1** provides a modification of such guidelines (see the Web site for additional information).

SUMMARY

In summary, PPD is a common, debilitating illness that has demonstrated distinction from major depression in research, despite categorization under major depression in the *DSM-5*. The risk factors associated with PPD span demographic, obstetric, psychiatric, and psychosocial variables. Predictors of PPD have been replicated in multiple studies and examined in multiple metaanalyses. As recommended by national standards, screening is of utmost importance in early detection of PPD in order to facilitate referral for treatment and ongoing monitoring. Consequences of untreated PPD for the mother range from social isolation to suicide, and consequences for the infant and family unit persist throughout child development. Treatment of PPD may include psychotherapy approaches, such as CBT, IPT, or listening visits. Medication treatment of PPD may include SSRI or newly approved brexanolone. Although PPD poses substantial risk for a mother and infant, early identification of risk for development of PPD, ongoing screening, and appropriate referrals for treatment may limit the adverse sequelae of the syndrome and thus promote lifelong maternal and familial health.

System recommendations include the following:
1. Ensure that all women are screened at least once for depression during both pregnancy and the postpartum period,
2. Educate providers on risk factors and screening tools,
3. Optimize detection of risk factors and symptoms,
4. Expedite referral and treatment,
5. Promptly identify suicidal behavior and refer for psychiatric intervention,
6. Discuss the impact of pregnancy on preexisting mental health conditions, including prior PPD, during preconception and prenatal care.

DISCLOSURE

E.B. Kroska has no competing interests to report. Z.N. Stowe has received research support and consultation honorarium from GlaxoSmithKline, Pfizer, and Wyeth Corporations and received speakers honoraria from these companies and Eli Lilly and Forest Corporations, but none of these relationships since 2008. He has received clinical trial support from Janssen Pharmaceuticals and Sage Therapeutics in the past 24 months and has received salary and research support from the National Institutes of Health and the Centers for Disease Control and Prevention.

REFERENCES

1. O'Hara MW. Postpartum depression: what we know. J Clin Psychol 2009;65: 1258–69.
2. O'Connor E, Senger CA, Henninger ML, et al. Interventions to prevent perinatal depression. JAMA 2019;321(6):588.
3. Curry SJ, Krist AH, Owens DK, et al. Interventions to prevent perinatal depression. JAMA 2019;321(6):580.
4. American Psychiatric Association. Diagnostic and statistical manual of mental disorders. 5th edition. Arlington (VA): American Psychiatric Association; 2013.
5. O'Hara MW, Schlechte JA, Lewis DA, et al. Prospective study of postpartum blues: biologic and psychosocial factors. Arch Gen Psychiatry 1991;48(9):801–6.
6. Heron J, McGuinness M, Blackmore ER, et al. Early postpartum symptoms in puerperal psychosis. BJOG 2008;115(3):348–53.
7. Ross LE, Gilbert Evans SE, Sellers EM, et al. Measurement issues in postpartum depression part 1: anxiety as a feature of postpartum depression. Arch Womens Ment Health 2003;6:51–7.
8. Miller ML, O'Hara MW. Obsessive-compulsive symptoms, intrusive thoughts and depressive symptoms: a longitudinal study examining relation to maternal responsiveness. J Reprod Infant Psychol 2019. https://doi.org/10.1080/02646838.2019.1652255.
9. O'Hara MW, Swain AM. Rates and risk of postpartum depression—a meta-analysis. Int Rev Psychiatry 1996;8(1):37–54.
10. Gavin NI, Gaynes BN, Lohr KN, et al. Perinatal depression: a systematic review of prevalence and incidence. Obstet Gynecol 2005;106(5, Part 1):1071–83.
11. Shorey S, Yin C, Chee I, et al. Prevalence and incidence of postpartum depression among healthy mothers: a systematic review and meta-analysis. J Psychiatr Res 2018;104:235–48.
12. Hahn-Holbrook J, Cornwell-Hinrichs T, Anaya I. Economic and health predictors of national postpartum depression prevalence: a systematic review, meta-analysis, and meta-regression of 291 studies from 56 countries. Front Psychiatry 2018;8. https://doi.org/10.3389/fpsyt.2017.00248.
13. O'Hara MW, Zekoski EM, Philipps LH, et al. Controlled prospective study of postpartum mood disorders: comparison of childbearing and nonchildbearing women. J Abnorm Psychol 1990;99(1):3–15.
14. Silverman ME, Reichenberg A, Lichtenstein P, et al. Is depression more likely following childbirth? A population-based study. Arch Womens Ment Health 2019;22(2):253–8.
15. Vesga-López O, Blanco C, Keyes K, et al. Psychiatric disorders in pregnant and postpartum women in the United States. Arch Gen Psychiatry 2008;65(7):805–15.

16. Eberhard-Gran M, Eskild A, Tambs K, et al. Depression in postpartum and non-postpartum women: prevalence and risk factors. Acta Psychiatr Scand 2002; 106(6):426–33.
17. Davé S, Petersen I, Sherr L, et al. Incidence of maternal and paternal depression in primary care: a cohort study using a primary care database. Arch Pediatr Adolesc Med 2010;164(11):1038–44.
18. Munk-Olsen T, Laursen TM, Pedersen CB, et al. New parents and mental disorders: a population-based register study. J Am Med Assoc 2006;296(21):2582–9.
19. Merkitch KG, Jonas KG, O'Hara MW. Modeling trait depression amplifies the effect of childbearing on postpartum depression. J Affect Disord 2017;223:69–75.
20. Viktorin A, Meltzer-Brody S, Kuja-Halkola R, et al. Heritability of perinatal depression and genetic overlap with nonperinatal depression. Am J Psychiatry 2016; 173:158–65.
21. Silverman ME, Reichenberg A, Savitz DA, et al. The risk factors for postpartum depression: a population-based study. Depress Anxiety 2017;34(2):178–87.
22. Azami M, Badfar G, Soleymani A, et al. The association between gestational diabetes and postpartum depression: a systematic review and meta-analysis. Diabetes Res Clin Pract 2019;149:147–55.
23. Hannah P, Adams D, Lee A, et al. Links between early post-partum mood and post-natal depression. Br J Psychiatry 1992;160:777–80.
24. Miller ML, Kroska EB, Grekin R. Immediate postpartum mood assessment and postpartum depressive symptoms. J Affect Disord 2017;207:69–75.
25. Siu AL, Bibbins-Domingo K, Grossman DC, et al. Screening for depression in adults: US preventive services task force recommendation statement. JAMA 2016;315(4):380–7.
26. Cox JL, Holden JM, Sagovsky R. Detection of postnatal depression: development of the 10-item Edinburgh postnatal depression scale. Br J Psychiatry 1987; 150(6):782–6.
27. Jairaj C, Fitzsimons CM, McAuliffe FM, et al. A population survey of prevalence rates of antenatal depression in the Irish obstetric services using the Edinburgh Postnatal Depression Scale (EPDS). Arch Womens Ment Health 2019;22(3): 349–55.
28. Kroenke K, Spitzer RL, Williams JBW. The PHQ-9: validity of a brief depression severity measure. J Gen Intern Med 2001;16(9):606–13.
29. Beck AT, Steer RA, Carbin MG. Psychometric properties of the Beck Depression Inventory: twenty-five years of evaluation. Clin Psychol Rev 1988;8(1):77–100.
30. Goodman SH, Gotlib IH. Risk for psychopathology in the children of depressed mothers: a developmental model for understanding mechanisms of transmission. Psychol Rev 1999;106(3):458–90.
31. Kersten-Alvarez LE, Hosman CMH, Riksen-Walraven JM, et al. Early school outcomes for children of postpartum depressed mothers: comparison with a community sample. Child Psychiatry Hum Dev 2012;43(2):201–18.
32. Murray L. The impact of postnatal depression on infant development. J Child Psychol Psychiatry 1992;33(3):543–61.
33. Grace SL, Evindar A, Stewart DE. The effect of postpartum depression on child cognitive development and behavior: a review and critical analysis of the literature. Arch Womens Ment Health 2003;6(4):263–74.
34. Sinclair D, Murray L. Effects of postnatal depression on children's adjustment to school: teacher's reports. Br J Psychiatry 1998;172:58–63.
35. Wisner KL, Chambers C, Sit DKY. Postpartum depression: a major public health problem. JAMA 2006;296(21):2616.

36. Meltzer-Brody S, Stuebe A. The long-term psychiatric and medical prognosis of perinatal mental illness. Best Pract Res Clin Obstet Gynaecol 2014;28(1):49–60.

37. Lindahl V, Pearson JL, Colpe L. Prevalence of suicidality during pregnancy and the postpartum. Arch Womens Ment Health 2005;8(2):77–87.

38. Field T. Postpartum depression effects on early interactions, parenting, and safety practices: a review. Infant Behav Dev 2010;33(1):1–6.

39. Goodman JH. Influences of maternal postpartum depression on fathers and on father-infant interaction. Infant Ment Health J 2008;29(6):624–43.

40. Letourneau NL, Dennis C-L, Benzies K, et al. Postpartum depression is a family affair: addressing the impact on mothers, fathers, and children. Issues Ment Health Nurs 2012;33(7):445–57.

41. Dennis C-L, Chung-Lee L. Postpartum depression help-seeking barriers and maternal treatment preferences: a qualitative systematic review. Birth 2006; 33(4):323–31.

42. Huang L, Zhao Y, Qiang C, et al. Is cognitive behavioral therapy a better choice for women with postnatal depression? A systematic review and meta-analysis. PLoS One 2018;13(10):e0205243.

43. Hayes SC. Acceptance and commitment therapy, relational frame theory, and the third wave of behavioral and cognitive therapies. Behav Ther 2004;35(4):639–65.

44. O'Hara MW, Stuart S, Gorman LL, et al. Efficacy of interpersonal psychotherapy for postpartum depression. Arch Gen Psychiatry 2000;57(11):1039–45.

45. Klier CM, Muzik M, Rosenblum KL, et al. Interpersonal psychotherapy adapted for the group setting in the treatment of postpartum depression. J Psychother Pract Res 2001;10(2):124–31.

46. Sockol LE, Epperson CN, Barber JP. Preventing postpartum depression: a meta-analytic review. Clin Psychol Rev 2013;33:1205–17.

47. Glavin K, Smith L, Sørum R, et al. Supportive counselling by public health nurses for women with postpartum depression. J Adv Nurs 2010;66(6):1317–27.

48. Holden JM, Sagovsky R, Cox JL. Counselling in a general practice setting: controlled study of home visitor intervention in treatment of postnatal depression. BMJ 1989;298:223–6.

49. Morrell CJ, Ricketts T, Tudor K, et al. Training health visitors in cognitive behavioural and person-centred approaches for depression in postnatal women as part of a cluster randomised trial and economic evaluation in primary care: the PoNDER trial. Prim Health Care Res Dev 2011;11–20. https://doi.org/10.1017/S1463423610000344.

50. Segre LS, Stasik SM, O'hara MW, et al. Listening visits: an evaluation of the effectiveness and acceptability of a home-based depression treatment. Psychother Res 2010;20(6):712–21.

51. Wisner KL, Peindl KS, Gigliotti TV. Tricyclics vs SSRIs for postpartum depression. Arch Womens Ment Health 1998;1(4):189–91.

52. Stowe ZN, Casarella J, Landry J, et al. Sertraline in the treatment of women with postpartum major depression. Depression 1995;3(1–2):49–55.

53. Hantsoo L, Ward-O'Brien D, Czarkowski KA, et al. A randomized, placebo-controlled, double-blind trial of sertraline for postpartum depression. Psychopharmacology (Berl) 2014;231(5):939–48.

54. Milgrom J, Gemmill AW, Ericksen J, et al. Treatment of postnatal depression with cognitive behavioural therapy, sertraline and combination therapy: a randomised controlled trial. Aust N Z J Psychiatry 2015;49(3):236–45.

55. Appleby L, Warner R, Whitton A, et al. A controlled study of fluoxetine and cognitive-behavioural counselling in the treatment of postnatal depression. Br Med J 1997;314(7085):932–6.
56. Misri S, Reebye P, Corral M, et al. The use of paroxetine and cognitive-behavioral therapy in postpartum depression and anxiety. J Clin Psychiatry 2004;65(9): 1236–41.
57. Yonkers KA, Lin H, Howell HB, et al. Pharmacologic treatment of postpartum women with new-onset major depressive disorder: a randomized controlled trial with paroxetine. J Clin Psychiatry 2008;69(4):659–65.
58. Suri R, Burt VK, Altshuler LL, et al. Fluvoxamine for postpartum depression. Am J Psychiatry 2001;158(10):1739–40. https://doi.org/10.1176/appi.ajp.158.10.1739.
59. Misri S, Abizadeh J, Albert G, et al. Restoration of functionality in postpartum depressed mothers. J Clin Psychopharmacol 2012;32(5):729–32.
60. Cohen LS, Viguera AC, Bouffard SM, et al. Venlafaxine in the treatment of postpartum depression. J Clin Psychiatry 2001;62(8):592–6.
61. Stowe ZN, Hostetter AL, Owens MJ, et al. The pharmacokinetics of sertraline excretion into human breast milk: determinants of infant serum concentrations. J Clin Psychiatry 2003;64(1):73–80.
62. Nonacs RM, Soares CN, Viguera AC, et al. Bupropion SR for the treatment of postpartum depression: a pilot study. Int J Neuropsychopharmacol 2005;8(3): 445–9.
63. Suri R, Burt VK, Altshuler LL. Nefazodone for the treatment of postpartum depression. Arch Womens Ment Health 2005;8:55–6.
64. Meltzer-Brody S, Colquhoun H, Riesenberg R, et al. Brexanolone injection in postpartum depression: two multicentre, double-blind, randomised, placebo-controlled, phase 3 trials. Lancet 2018;392(1058–1070):1058–70.
65. Kanes S, Colquhoun H, Gunduz-Bruce H, et al. Brexanolone (SAGE-547 injection) in post-partum depression: a randomised controlled trial. Lancet 2017; 390(10093):480–9.
66. Werner E, Miller M, Osborne LM, et al. Preventing postpartum depression: review and recommendations. Arch Womens Ment Health 2015;18(1):41–60.
67. Wisner KL, Perel JM, Peindl KS, et al. Prevention of postpartum depression: a pilot randomized clinical trial. Am J Psychiatry 2004;161(7):1290–2.
68. Robertson E, Grace S, Wallington T, et al. Antenatal risk factors for postpartum depression: a synthesis of recent literature. Gen Hosp Psychiatry 2004;26(4): 289–95.
69. Beck CT. Predictors of postpartum depression: an update. Nurs Res 2001;50(5): 275–85.

Opioid Management in Pregnancy and Postpartum

Haywood L. Brown, MD

KEYWORDS

- Pregnancy • opioid use disorder • Postoperative pain management
- Opioid agonist maintenance

KEY POINTS

- Pregnant women with opioid use disorder present unique challenges for patients and providers throughout the perinatal period.
- Pain management during labor and for cesarean delivery should meet the needs of the patient and use evidence-based prescribing algorithms.
- Women on maintenance agonist therapy require coordinated management.
- Women with opioid use disorder are at significant risk for relapse, and postpartum follow-up is essential to decrease risk for relapse drug overdose and maternal mortality.

INTRODUCTION

The opioid epidemic in the United States has not bypassed the pregnant woman with opioid prescriptions, with opioid use significantly increasing over the past decade. Opioids are the most common illicit substance for which pregnancy women seek treatment.[1] The challenges of caring for pregnant and postpartum women with a history of opioid addiction and those on agonist maintenance therapy pose unique challenges for the women, providers, and health care teams. In 2007%, 22.8% of women enrolled in a Medicaid program in 46 states filled an opioid prescription during pregnancy.[2] The result of the rising use of opioids during pregnancy has led to an increase in neonatal abstinence syndrome (NAS), from 1.5 cases per 1000 births in 1999 to 6.0 per 1000 hospital births in 2013.[3,4] Between 2004 and 2013, the incidence of NAS per 1000 hospital births among rural infants increased from 1.2 to 7.5 and from 1.4 to 4.8 among urban infants.[5] In Tennessee, the rate of NAS in rural east Tennessee was 26.2 per 1000 births compared with 5.6 per 1000 births in the urban Nashville area.[6] With regard to states, NAS incidence was lowest in Hawaii, at 0.7 per 1000 births, compared with West Virginia, at 33.4 per 1000 births.[7] The cost for NAS and neonatal withdrawal treatment in the United States was estimated at approximately $1.5 billion in 2015.[3]

University of South Florida, 13101 Bruce B. Downs Drive, MDC, Tampa, FL 33612, USA
E-mail address: haywoodb@usf.edu

Obstet Gynecol Clin N Am 47 (2020) 421–427
https://doi.org/10.1016/j.ogc.2020.04.005
0889-8545/20/© 2020 Elsevier Inc. All rights reserved.

obgyn.theclinics.com

The rates of heroin use and prescription opioid–related overdose deaths are rising faster in women than men, in particular, women of reproductive age.[8] Between 2015 and 2016, the rate of overdose deaths among women rose 20%.[9] Furthermore, pregnancy-associated overdose deaths related to opioids also has seen a dramatic increase as a contributor to maternal mortality. Among all pregnancy-associated deaths, 11% to 20% were due to opioid overdose.[10] In a report by Schiff and colleagues,[11] overdose deaths were lowest in the third trimester (3.3/100000 person days) and then increased in the postpartum period, with the highest overdose rate 7 months to 12 months after delivery (12.3/100000 per days). The Texas Department of Health Services conducted an analysis of maternal deaths resulting from overdoses from 2012 to 2015. The risk for drug overdose maternal death was higher among white women, those women ages 40 years and older, those from urban counties, and those enrolled in Medicaid at the time of delivery. Of the 64 drug overdose deaths, 49 (77%) involved a combination of drugs; however, opioids, including heroin, accounted for 2 of the top 3 specific drugs identified in drug overdose maternal deaths.[12]

OPIOID USE DISORDER IN PREGNANCY

Opioid use disorder (OUD) can develop with repetitive use of any opioid, particularly for individuals with an underlying genetic vulnerability. OUD is characterized by chronic opioid use leading to tolerance, craving, and the inability to control use. Opioids are prescribed for pain and diminish the intensity of pain signals. It is the sense of euphoria, however, that occurs with opioid use that has led to significant increase in misuse over the past decade. OUD is a chronic condition and in 2016 was designated by the Surgeon General as a chronic neurologic disorder. The *Diagnostic and Statistical Manual of Mental Disorders* (Fifth Edition) outlines 11 main symptoms of OUD and defines the severity of OUD based on the number of recurring symptoms experienced within a 12-month period. Severity is defined as mild (2 to 3 symptoms), moderate (4 to 5 symptoms), or severe (6 or more symptoms).[13,14]

Opioid use in pregnancy has not showed an increased risk for birth defects after first-trimester exposure to oxycodone, propoxyphene, or merperidine.[15] The data on opioids and birth defects, however, are conflicting, with studies showing an increased risk for several birth defects with the use of opioids in the month prior to pregnancy and during the first trimester.[16]

Chronic opioid misuse and addiction during pregnancy are associated with inadequate prenatal care, fetal growth restriction, placental abruption, fetal death, preterm labor, and meconium passage in utero.[17] Pregnant women with untreated OUD often suffer co-occurring mental health conditions, including depression and posttraumatic stress, and engage in high risk activities, such as trading sex for drugs, thereby exposing themselves to sexually transmitted infections, violence, and incarceration.[18]

With regard to mental health disorders, approximately 30% of pregnant women enrolled in a substance use treatment program screened positive for moderate to severe depression and more than 40% reported symptoms of postpartum depression[19] and were at increased risk for polydrug use and abuse.[20]

Long-term use leads to physiologic dependence, which results in withdrawal on discontinuation. Symptoms of opioid withdrawal include generalized pain, muscle pain, nausea, diarrhea, sweating, rhinorrhea, tearing, dilated pupils, tremors, gooseflesh, restlessness, and anxiety. Short term opioids (eg heroin) lead to withdrawal symptoms within 4 hours to 6 hours of use, peak at 1 day to 3 days, and subside over 5 days to 7 days. Long-acting opioids, such as methadone, result in withdrawal within 24 hours to 36 hours of use and last for several weeks.[14]

PAIN MANAGEMENT POSTPARTUM

Opioids have been prescribed routinely for management of postcesarean pain and unfortunately for some women after vaginal delivery. One study indicated that 85.4% of women filled an opioid prescription after cesarean delivery. One in 300 women becomes dependent on opioids after a cesarean delivery.[21] Overprescribing has been common, and prescribing opioids after vaginal delivery should be exceedingly rare. Opioid prescribing after cesarean has been challenged in recent years based on data of actual number of doses used in the early postpartum period. For example, the average number of pills dispensed in the study, described previously, was 40; the median number of pills consumed was 20; and the average number of leftover pills was 15 and they were not properly disposed of.[22]

Cesarean delivery is one of the most common surgical procedures in the United States, and pain management is critical to recovery and care of the newborn. Perioperative care, including pain management, enhances recovery, quality of care, and patient satisfaction. Risk factors for persistent use of opioids after cesarean include receipt of a postoperative prescription, prescription size or number, concurrent pain diagnosis, other substance abuse disorder, and mood disorders.[22,23] The American College of Obstetricians and Gynecologists has recommendations for a stepwise approach to pain control based on the World Health Organization model.[23] For postoperative cesarean pain, this includes standard oral and parenteral analgesic, adjuvant acetaminophen, nonsteroidal anti-inflammatory drugs (NSAIDS), opioids, and opioids that are in combination formulations with acetaminophen or an NSAID.[23] Obviously, pain management begins with neuraxial opioids for postcesarean birth analgesia followed by additional analgesia once the effects of neuraxial opioid diminish.[23,24] Parenteral opioids or oral opioids should be reserved for treating breakthrough pain when combination neuraxial opioids and nonopioid adjuncts proved inadequate in controlling pain. The oral route is preferred for opioids and is just as effective as parenterally administered opioids.[25] Parenteral opioid should be reserved for those women who cannot tolerate oral medications. If parenteral opioids are used, patient-controlled analgesic is preferred for greater analgesic efficacy and patient satisfaction.[25,26]

A shared decision-making approach to postpartum discharge opioid prescribing can optimize pain control and at the same time reduced the number of pills prescribed and the number of unused opioid tablets that should be disposed of.[27,28]

Implementation of Enhanced Recovery after Surgery, which is a comprehensive, interdisciplinary protocol-based approach beginning in the preoperative period and extending into the postoperative period for cesarean delivery, has quickly gained acceptance in current perioperative management.[29]

Women with chronic pain disorders who use opioids require special attention with regard to pain management for labor, delivery, and postpartum. If available, these women should be managed in collaboration with specialist consultants in pain management, which typically include anesthesiologists, addiction medicine specialists, pain management specialists, pediatricians who have knowledge of ramifications of NAS and withdrawal expectations, behavioral medicine, obstetricians, and maternal fetal medicine subspecialists with expertise in chronic pain in pregnancy, and, most importantly, social services.

Pain management should include minimizing the use of opioids and nonopioid pharmacologic medications for postpartum pain.

For women with OUD who have scheduled or emergency cesarean delivery, postoperative neuraxial opioid is appropriate as with nonopioid women. Adjunctive methods should be considered to assist with postoperative pain control. For example, these women are potential candidates for local anesthetics delivered by wound infiltration[30] or transversus abdominis plane block, which involves using a blunt tip needle to inject 20 mL to 30 mL of a local anesthetic into the plane between the internal oblique and transversus abdominis muscles, targeting peripheral nerves innervating the lower abdomen.[31] Ketorolac also can be used at the end of the cesarean if not contraindicated.

Acetaminophen, intravenously or orally, can be used as a first-line treatment of postoperative pain for those women with OUD.

This management for postoperative pain should serve as a guideline for those with OUD and maintenance medications, methadone and buprenorphine.

MANAGEMENT OF WOMEN ON MAINTENANCE MEDICATION FOR OPIOID ADDICTION

Management of perinatal OUD has long included maintenance medications, historically with methadone and more recently with buprenorphine. Both opioid agonist pharmacotherapies used as medication-assisted treatment are efficacious for the management of perinatal OUD. Opioid agonist medication-assisted treatment not only prevents withdrawal but also reduces relapse risk, especially when combined with behavioral strategies that are included in an established addiction treatment program. Methadone is a full, mu-opioid receptor agonist that is dispensed daily through federally accredited opioid treatment programs. Buprenorphine is a partial mu-opioid receptor agonist and is administered in an office-based treatment setting and can be prescribed by providers, including obstetricians who have completed a training program and obtained a waiver through the Drug Enforcement Administration. Buprenorphine can be prescribed as a monotherapy (Subutex) or in combination with naloxone (Suboxone) and is self-administered. The advantage favoring buprenorphine is that the woman does not have to make daily office visits. Both are safe to use during pregnancy and there is no evidence that either buprenorphine or methadone causes birth defects. There is some evidence that women on buprenorphine have an associated reduced risk in severity of NAS.[32,33] Unfortunately, there are fewer qualified providers for medication-assisted treatment in rural communities, where needs for treatment programs and postpartum follow-up most often are a barrier in preventing relapse.

Management of labor, delivery, and postpartum pain for women on maintenance medication is similar to that for other postpartum women with OUD except for how maintenance medication is handled during the postpartum recovery period. Maintenance doses should be continued during labor and the intrapartum and immediate postpartum periods. Immediately postpartum, NSAIDS are highly effective, especially after vaginal delivery. An algorithm for postoperative pain for women on buprenorphine is shown in **Box 1**.

Shared decision making is important in postpartum pain management, particularly after hospital discharge. Pain management during the first 72 hours postpartum with regard to medications required to control pain can be used as a guide to prescribed medications after discharge. For patients on maintenance medication, the pain medication prescribed at discharge should be communicated to the outpatient opioid treatment program where the postpartum woman receives follow-up care.

Medication-assisted withdrawal or opioid detoxification during pregnancy and postpartum has proved successful for motivated patients with OUD. Results of a systematic review of 1126 pregnant women who underwent opioid detoxification showed

---

Box 1
Postoperative pain management for women on buprenorphine maintenance

First 2 hours postoperative (neuraxial analgesia)

Ketorolac scheduled around the clock

Maintenance buprenorphine in divided doses, 2 times to 3 times daily (if normally 8 mg/d, give 4 mg every 12 h)

Additional buprenorphine, 2 mg every 4 hours, as needed, for breakthrough pain, not to exceed a maximum of 30 mg/d

Intravenous or oral acetaminophen as alternative pain medication for those with OUD

Postoperative day 1, switch from Ketorolac to ibuprofen

Discharge postoperative day 3 with NSAIDs to follow-up with delivery and/or buprenorphine provider within the first 3 weeks postpartum

NO NARCOTICS

---

wide variability for success and concomitant illicit drug use.[34] Rates of relapse are lower for women who have longer tapering schedules and more intensive behavioral care over longer periods of time.[35] Shared decision making between patient and providers willing to support a woman's wishes for medication-assisted withdrawal, based on motivation to minimize the risk for NAS and achieving a long-term goal of freedom for maintenance therapy while balancing the life stressors that exist with maintaining sobriety and potential relapse, is critical in any model for success for these women. For these women, medication-assisted withdrawal should be provided under the supervision of those with expertise in addiction medicine.

Breastfeeding should be encouraged for women with OUD and those on medication-assisted maintenance who are stable on opioid agonist and not using illicit drugs. Minimal levels of methadone and buprenorphine appear in breast milk.

SUMMARY

Pregnant and postpartum women with OUD, with chronic pain disorders, who use opioids, and who participate in medication-assisted treatment programs require special support during pregnancy, especially in the postpartum period. Women with OUD are subjected to certain stigma that further complicates the management during pregnancy, labor, delivery, and postpartum. Postpartum is a particularly stressful and vulnerable period for women with OUD, including access to quality and continuity of care, concerns for a newborn with NAS who is likely still under neonatal intensive care, and potential child custody and legal issues. These women also are at higher risk for relapse and drug overdose and death.[11] Pregnancy and postpartum provide an opportunity for patients and obstetric care providers to support and advocate for women with OUD and assist them in maintaining positive health behaviors as well as shared decision making in contraceptive counseling and choices. A supportive team approach to care without stigmatization for women with OUD lessens the risk for perinatal morbidity and the potential for mortality. This continuum of care must encompass the prenatal period, intrapartum period, and, most importantly, postpartum follow-up.

DISCLOSURE

None.

REFERENCES

1. Jumah NA. Rural, pregnant and opioid dependent: a systematic review. Subst Abuse 2016;10(Suppl 1):35–41.
2. Desai RJ, Hernandez-Diaz S, Bateman BT, et al. Increase in prescription opioid use during pregnancy among Medicaid enrolled women. Obstet Gynecol 2014; 123:997–1002.
3. Patrick SW, Davis MM, Lehman CU, et al. Increasing incidence and geographic distribution of neonatal abstinence syndrome: United States 2009 to 2012. J Perinatal 2015;35:650–5.
4. Sanlorenzo LA, Stark AR, Patrick SW. Neonatal abstinence syndrome: An update. Curr Opin Pediatr 2018;30(2):182–6.
5. Villapiano NG, Winkelman TA, Kozhimannil KD, et al. rural and urban differences in neonatal abstinence syndrome and maternal opioid use. 2004 to 2013. JAMA Pediatr 2017;171(2):194–6.
6. Miller A, McDonald M, Warren MD. Neonatal Abstinence syndrome surveillance annual report. 2016. Available at: https://www.tn.gov/assets/entities/health/attachments?NAS_Annual _report_2016_Final.pdf. Accessed March 24, 2020.
7. Ko JY, Patrick SW, Tong VT, et al. Incidence of Neonatal Abstinence Syndrome – 28 States. 1999-2013. MMWR Morb Mortal Wkly Rep 2016;65(31):799–802.
8. Cicero TK, Eos S, Sirratt JL, et al. The changing face of heroin use in the United States: a retrospective analysis of the past 50 years. JAMA psychiatry 2014; 71(7):821–6.
9. US Opioid Crisis: Addressing maternal and infant health. Division of Reproductive health, National Center for Chronic Disease Prevention and Heath Promotion. Available at: www.cdc.gov/reproductivehealth/opioid-use-disorder-pregnancy/index.html.
10. Metz TD, Rovener P, Hoffman MC, et al. Maternal deaths from suicide and overdose in Colorado, 2004-2012. Obstet Gynecol 2016;128(6):1233–40.
11. Schiff DM, Nielson T, Terplan M, et al. Fatal and nonfatal overdose among pregnancy and postpartum women in Massachusetts. Obstet Gynecol 2018;132(2):466–74.
12. Texas Health and Human Services/Texas Department of State Health Services. The role of opioid overdoses in confirmed maternal death 2012-2016. 2017. Available at: https://www.dshs.texas.gov/mch/pdf/Confirmed -Maternal-Deaths-Due to Drug-Overdose.pdf. Accessed March 23, 2020.
13. American Psychiatric Association. Diagnostic and statistical manual of mental disorders. 5th edition. Arlington (VA): APA; 2013.
14. Opioid use and opioid use disorder in pregnancy. Committee Opinion No. 711. American College of Obstetricians and Gynecologist. Obstet Gynecol 2017;130:e81-94.(Reaffirmed 2019)
15. Jick H, Holmes LB, KJuner JR, et al. First-trimester drug use and congenital disorders. JAMA 1981;246:343–6.
16. Broussard CS, Rasmussen SA, Reefhuis J, et al. Maternal treatment with opioid analgesics and risk for birth defects. National Birth Defects Prevention Study. Am J Obstet Gynecol 2011;204:314.e1-11.
17. Center for Substance Abuse Treatment. Medication-assisted treatment for opioid addiction during pregnancy. In: Medication assisted treatment for opioid addiction in opioid treatment programs. Treatment improvement protocol (TIP Series, No. 43). Rockville (MD): Substance Abuse and Mental Health Services Administration; 2005. p. 211–24.

18. Ecker J, Abhamad A, Hill W, et al. Substance use disorders in pregnancy: clinical, ethical, and research imperatives of the opioid epidemic: a report of a joint workshop of the Society for Maternal Fetal medicine, American College of Obstetricians and Gynecologists, and American Society of Addiction Medicine, SMFM Special Report. Am J Obstet Gynecol 2019;B5–28.
19. Holbrook A, Kaltenbach K. Co-occurring psychiatric symptoms in opioid-dependent women: the prevalence of antenatal and postnatal depression. Am J Drug Alcohol Abuse 2012;38:575–9.
20. Jones HE, Heil ISH, O'Grady KE, et al. Smoking in pregnant women screened for an opioid agonist medication study compared to related pregnant and non-pregnant patient samples. Am J Drug Alcohol Abuse 2009;35:375–80.
21. Bateman BT, Franklin JM, Bykov K, et al. Persistent opioid use following cesarean delivery: patterns and predictors among opioid-naïve women. Am J Obstet Gynecol 2016;215:353.e1-18.
22. Bateman BT, Cole NM, Maeda A, et al. Patterns of opioid prescription and use after cesarean delivery. Obstet Gynecol 2017;130:29–35.
23. American College of Obstetricians and Gynecologists. Postpartum pain management. ACOG Committee opinion no. 742. Obstet Gynecol 2018;132:e35–43.
24. Sutton CD, Carvalho B. Optimal pain management after cesarean delivery. Anesthesiol Clin 2017;35:107–24.
25. Davis KM, Esposito MA, Meyer BA. Oral analgesia compared with intravenous patient-controlled analgesia for pain after cesarean delivery: a randomized controlled trial. Am J Obstet Gynecol 2006;194:967–71.
26. McNicol ED, Ferguson MC, Hudcova J. Patient controlled opioid analgesia versus non-patient controlled opioid analgesia for postoperative pain. Cochrane Database Syst Rev 2015;(6):CD003348.
27. Prabhu M, McQuaid-Hanson E, Hopp S, et al. A shared decision-making intervention to guide opioid prescribing after cesarean delivery. Obstet Gynecol 2017;130:42–6.
28. Howard R, Wajee J, Burmmett C, et al. Reduction in opioid prescribing through evidence-based prescribing guidelines. JAMA Surg 2018;153:132, 285–7.
29. Peahjl AF, Smith R, Johnson TRB, et al. Better late than never: Why obstetricians must implement enhanced recovery after cesarean. Am J Obstet Gynecol 2019;221:117–23.
30. Lavand'homme PM, Roelants F, Waterloos H, et al. Postoperative analgesic effects of continuous wound infiltration with diclofenac after elective cesarean delivery. Anesthesiology 2007;106:1220–5.
31. Eslamian L, Jalili Z, Jamal A, et al. Transversus abdominis plane block reduces postoperative pain intensity and analgesic consumption in elective cesarean delivery under general anesthesia. J Anesth 2012;26:334–8.
32. Jones HE, Kaltenbach K, Heil SH, et al. Neonatal abstinence syndrome after methadone or buprenorphine exposure. N Engl J Med 2010;363:2320–31.
33. Noomohammadi A, Forinash A, Yancey A, et al. Buprenorphine versus methadone for opioid dependence in pregnancy. Ann Pharmacother 2016;50:666–72.
34. Terplan M, Laird HJ, Hand DJ, et al. Opioid detoxification during pregnancy. A systematic review. Obstet Gynecol 2018;131:803–14.
35. Bell J, Towers CV, Hennessay MD, et al. Detoxification from opiate drugs during pregnancy. Am J Obstet Gynecol 2016;15(3):374.e1-6.

Reducing Cesarean Delivery Surgical Site Complications

Margaret S. Villers, MD, MSCR

KEYWORDS

- Cesarean delivery • Surgical site infection • Wound complication

KEY POINTS

- Antibiotic prophylaxis before surgery and adding azithromycin will decrease infectious complications for labor patients.
- Surgeons should use Pfannenstiel incisions, meticulous surgical techniques, including closure of subcutaneous tissue, and subcuticular suture to decrease wound complications.
- Preoperative vaginal cleansing is a new technique to reduce the risk of endometritis.
- Dehiscence is associated with significant risk for morbidity and mortality and increased cost of care.

Women with postpartum cesarean delivery (CD) surgical site infections (SSI) or wound complications experience significant disruptions during the postpartum period. Approximately 10% of women with a CD experience a wound complication.[1,2] Of women who experience a postpartum hospital readmission, 39% were due to a postpartum CD SSI.[3] Unfortunately, most studies do not capture the number of women diagnosed with an SSI who are treated as an outpatient. Not all wound complications are associated with infection. Postcesarean wound complications also include seromas and hematomas. These complications may also require inpatient hospitalization and outpatient treatment that can disrupt recovery. However, it is difficult to characterize these wound complications because of varying definitions. Women may require multiple outpatient visits to their physician for treatment of cellulitis, seroma, hematoma, or other complications. Home health care follow-up may extend for several weeks depending on availability of such services.

There are no published data on the impact that CD wound complications have on the maternal postpartum recovery. It can be theorized that women may discontinue breastfeeding sooner or experience postpartum depression. Likely, these women are treated with antibiotics and are given prescriptions for multiple pain medications, including ongoing prescriptions for opioids. Studies on health care costs focus solely

Maternal-Fetal Medicine, Mary Washington Medical Group, 1300 Hospital Drive #200, Fredericksburg, VA 22401, USA
E-mail address: margaret.villers@mwhc.com

Obstet Gynecol Clin N Am 47 (2020) 429–437
https://doi.org/10.1016/j.ogc.2020.04.006
0889-8545/20/© 2020 Elsevier Inc. All rights reserved.

obgyn.theclinics.com

on hospital costs and costs directly attributable to infection.[4] Those costs do not capture time lost from work for follow-up physician visits, out-of-pocket medical expenses, care needed for the newborn, or emotional distress.

The best method to decrease postpartum SSI is prevention. Today, pregnant women are more likely to have multiple medical conditions, including diabetes and hypertension. In addition, the degree of obesity has increased markedly in the past few years.[5] Evidence suggests that obesity is associated with postoperative morbidity, including wound complications.[6] Obesity is theorized to impact wound healing through various mechanisms, including inherent anatomic features of adipose tissue, vascular insufficiencies, cellular and compositions modifications, oxidative stress, alterations in immune mediators, and nutritional deficiencies.[7] These factors are not modifiable at time of delivery, which means evidence-based best practices surrounding CD must be adopted.

Recently, the focus on enhanced recovery after surgery (ERAS) has been adapted to CD and adopted by obstetricians. ERAS represents evidence-based best practices, and it also focuses on shortening the stay after delivery and optimizing patient experience.[8,9] Similarly, published studies of a bundled approach to surgical techniques and perioperative interventions applied to cesarean deliveries have demonstrated unique implementation methods focused on decreasing the CD SSI rate.[10,11] Unfortunately, despite improvements in preoperative and surgical techniques, the CD wound complication rate remains high.

Many interventions to reduce SSI, including hair clippers, have been widely adopted. The objective of this article is not to perform an exhaustive review of all methods of reducing CD SSI or wound complication. Instead, the goal is to focus on debated evidence-based interventions that demonstrate the most benefit and the impact wound complications have on maternal morbidity and recovery.

PREOPERATIVE ANTIMICROBIAL PROPHYLAXIS

The American College of Obstetricians and Gynecologists (ACOG) recommends antibiotic prophylaxis administered within 60 minutes of skin incision.[12] Cefazolin, a first-generation cephalosporin, is recommended as the first-line antibiotic of choice because it is effective against most bacteria that are present at time of delivery. Weight-based dosing is common in most hospitals despite limited evidence of increased efficacy.[13]

For women with a significant allergy to penicillin or cephalosporin, clindamycin with an aminoglycoside, usually gentamycin, is acceptable. There are limited data on the effectiveness of clindamycin and gentamycin to reduce infectious complications after surgery.

Recently, a large randomized trial demonstrated reduction in the number of wound infections when azithromycin was added to the routine antibiotic regimen in laboring women. The addition of azithromycin reduced the incidence of wound infections from 6.6% to 2.4% (relative risk [RR]: 0.35; 95% confidence interval [CI]: 0.22–0.56). The addition of azithromycin to prevent wound infections also resulted in a reduction of unscheduled clinic visits, emergency room visits, and readmissions.[2]

Determining choice of appropriate antibiotics can be challenging, because a penicillin or cephalosporin allergy is documented in up to 20% of patients.[14] The actual type of allergic reaction is rarely documented despite the increase of electronic medical records.[15] A true penicillin allergy is a type 1 hypersensitivity reaction that is manifested as immediate hives, angioedema, or anaphylaxis. Few women with a documented penicillin allergy actually have a severe penicillin allergy.[14]

When a woman reports an allergy to penicillin, beta-lactam antibiotics are avoided, and non-beta-lactam antibiotics, such as clindamycin and gentamycin, are used. A recent cohort study demonstrated that of women who received non-beta-lactam antibiotics, 15% were diagnosed with an SSI compared with 7% who received a beta-lactam antibiotic.[16] This finding suggests that clindamycin and gentamycin, non-beta-lactam antibiotics, may not provide adequate antimicrobial coverage for prevention of infectious morbidity after CD.[16] Women without a severe penicillin reaction should be treated with cefazolin per ACOG guidelines.[12] Penicillin skin testing is gaining wider acceptance to determine if women have true penicillin allergies. Penicillin skin testing allows for a more accurate evaluation of antimicrobial allergies and use of more effective antibiotics.

PREOPERATIVE PREPARATION

Preoperative skin cleansing, also referred to as skin prepping, is recommended before surgery to reduce infectious organisms on the skin. Several preparation techniques and solutions have been evaluated over the decades, and surgical scholars debate the timing of the preparation as well as whether the solution should be allowed to dry before making the incision. Currently, the best evidence supports chlorhexidine (CHG) alcohol as the preferred skin preparation solution recommended by most experts and widely used in many hospitals.[17] However, there appears to be no difference between using povidone iodine or CHG alcohol for reduction of SSI.[18,19] The mechanical cleansing of the skin likely contributes most to pathogen reduction. Therefore, skin preparation techniques play as significant a role as the choice of solution used in cleansing the skin before incision.

Preoperative bathing is commonly recommended to reduce infections in general surgery patients. There have been no studies of preoperative bathing before CD. Many CDs performed nonelectively, which precludes planned bathing. CHG wipes have been incorporated into infectious reduction bundles to reduce skin flora.[10,20] The wipes are used directly on the abdomen up to 6 hours before surgery. Unfortunately, no trials have been performed to determine the effect of CHG wipes.

CD infections can be caused by bacteria originating from the skin or the vagina. Preoperative vaginal cleansing has been shown to decrease endometritis in women who were laboring or had ruptured membranes.[21] A Cochrane Review of vaginal preparation before surgery demonstrated a reduced incidence of endometritis in women undergoing CD. The greatest reduction occurred in women with ruptured membranes.[22] Both povidone iodine and CHG have been used as surgical skin preparations in vaginal surgery. CHG has greater efficacy then povidone iodine on reduction of bacterial counts in the vagina. Studies regarding vagina preparation before CD have focused on use of povidone iodine because of Food and Drug Administration warning of utilization of CHG on mucous membranes. CHG may be superior to povidone iodine in the vagina because povidone iodine is inactive in the presence of blood.[23] Blood in the vagina occurs during all deliveries, including CDs. During a CD, blood is expressed from the uterus into the vagina. CHG with low concentrations of alcohol can be safely used off-label.[12] Several trials of vaginal cleansing performed during CD have demonstrated a reduction of SSIs in women undergoing CD regardless of solution used.

SURGICAL TECHNIQUE

The Pfannenstiel incision is most commonly used for CD even for women with obesity. However, surgeons continue to debate whether Pfannenstiel or vertical skin incision is associated with lower risk for wound complications in the morbidly obese woman with pannus. Vertical incisions are associated with a 2-fold increase in postoperative infections compared with Pfannenstiel incisions in women undergoing CD during labor.[24] Morbidly obese women have a significantly higher rate of wound infection when a vertical incision is used rather than a sub–pannus transverse incision.[25,26]

A Cochrane Review compared the Joel-Cohen incision with Pfannenstiel incision and showed an overall 65% reduction in postoperative febrile morbidity (RR: 0.35; 95% CI: 0.14–0.87; P = .23) with the Joel-Cohen incision. Other benefits from the Joel-Cohen technique included a lower need for postoperative analgesia and lower blood loss.[27,28] The CORONIS trial is a multicentered, unmasked randomized controlled trial from 19 institutions that assessed the effect of 5 elements of the cesarean technique in maternal and neonatal outcomes. Blunt versus sharp abdominal entry was examined as one of the variables and did not demonstrate a significant difference in febrile morbidity or wound complications between the groups.[29]

SKIN CLOSURE

Published studies have focused on specific surgical techniques to reduce the incidence of SSI. Closure of the subcutaneous space is recommended if there is greater than 2 cm of tissue thickness.[30] Closure of the subcutaneous space compared with nonclosure is associated with a significant decrease in wound separation, seroma, as well as wound infection.[31]

Skin closure with sutures has gained wide acceptance as the preferred skin closure method because it reduces the risk of wound separation and other complications.[32,33] A metaanalysis concluded that staple closure is associated with a 2-fold increase of wound infection and separation compared with subcuticular sutures.[33] A multicentered randomized controlled trial found a 57% decrease in the incidence of wound complications, including wound infection, with suture closure compared with staples (4.9% compared with 10.6%; odds ratio [OR]; 0.43; 95% CI: 0.23–0.78).[32] Wound separations are significantly lower for suture closure compared with staples: 7.4% versus 1.6% (OR: 0.2; 95% CI: 0.07–0.51).[34]

Some communities prefer the use of absorbable subcuticular staples. Unfortunately, there are limited data about the use of subcuticular staples. One published cohort study demonstrated comparable wound complication rates with subcuticular staples and subcuticular sutures. Both methods had a lower rate of wound complications than traditional skin staples.[35] Subcuticular staple closure may be an acceptable alternative to subcuticular suture closure.

NEGATIVE PRESSURE WOUND THERAPY

Negative pressure wound therapy (NPWT) dressings have been theorized to reduced SSIs as well as seromas or hematomas. Several mechanisms have been proposed as an explanation for why NPWT promotes wound healing. The most common mechanisms include removal of extracellular fluid, release of cytokines and inflammatory factors, and improvement of tissue oxygenation.[36] Most obviously, NPWT also serves as a physical barrier; it keeps the incision covered and may prevent exposure to microbes.

No trial has conclusively proved that NPWT reduces the incidence of CD wound complication or infection in the general population. The cost of NPWT is substantial and adds to the cost of care. A cost-effectiveness analysis demonstrated that NPWT is not cost-beneficial in populations at low risk for CD SSI.[37] However, NPWT may reduce the SSIs in certain subsets of women with high-risk factors, including obesity.[38,39] A metaanalysis demonstrated a 55% reduction of SSI and other wound complications with the use of NPWT in a population of obese women.[38] A randomized controlled trial of women with a body mass index more than 30 demonstrated a 50% RR for SSI.[39]

COMPLICATED SURGICAL SITE INFECTIONS

Abdominal wound dehiscence ultimately results in prolonged wound healing depending on management of the initial wound disruptions. The mortality for abdominal laparotomy dehiscence has been reported to be as high as 45% even though most obstetric patients are for the most part young and otherwise healthy except for the high rate of obesity in the young obstetric population.[40] Significant wound complications should be immediately opened and explored. Wound complications must be carefully inspected for fascia disruption and signs of necrotizing fasciitis (NF). Fascial disruptions require immediate surgical management to decrease risk for morbidity.

NF is a severe infection involving the skin, subcutaneous tissue, and superficial fascia, which often has a fulminant course and a potentially lethal outcome. It is a rare infection with an estimated incidence of 0.4 per 100,000 in the general population and a mortality of up to 34%. Methicillin-resistant *Staphylococcus aureus* has been implicated in up to a third of cases.[40,41] Treatment of NF with antibiotics plays an irreplaceable role in management; however, surgical intervention is the mainstay of management and should be done promptly. Antibiotic therapy without debridement is associated with a mortality approaching 100%.[42]

Management of wound dehiscence has evolved over the last couple of decades with clinical management primarily focused on debridement followed by wound vacuum and home wound care and healing by secondary intent. Vacuum-assisted wound closure (VAC) may be considered medically appropriate in the home setting to promote the closure of chronic wounds. It is used as an adjunct therapy or as an alternative to surgery. Depending on the size of the wound and prolonged visiting home nursing for VAC changing, the cost of care can be quite significant. Evidence-based guidelines for management of postoperative wound dehiscence after CD are limited and thereby have led to wide variations in management strategies.[43] Traditional management relied on debridement followed by wet to dry dressing and healing by secondary intention. Traditional management methods have largely been replaced by home wound vacuum management, which prolongs care and continues to impact daily living. Previous reports described debridement, following and a short period of

Table 1
Summary of recommendations to reduce cesarean delivery surgical site complications

Intervention	
Antimicrobial prophylaxis	Cefazolin is first line for antimicrobial prophylaxis
	Add azithromycin to standard prophylaxis when CD is performed in labor
	Screen carefully for penicillin allergies
Skin preparation	CHG alcohol is widely used in most hospitals
	Skin preparation technique is as important as choice of solution
	Use of CHG wipes should be investigated for nonelective CD
	Vaginal cleansing with CHG or povidone iodine decreases endometritis
Surgical technique	Transverse skin incisions are associated with a lower risk of SSIs
	The Joel-Cohen technique may provide additional benefits
Skin closure	Subcutaneous tissue should be reapproximated if it is >2 cm thick
	Absorbable sutures reduce the risk of wound complications
NPWT	Used in morbidly obese women, NPWT significantly reduces wound infections

granulation and reclosure.[44,45] A recent report focused on debridement and immediate reclosure without a period of granulation as a management option for surgical site dehiscence.[46] The investigators describe complete healing with a median healing time of 20 days and avoidance of prolonged periods of disability and frequent follow-up office visits and home care visits of wound care management with healing by secondary intention.

SUMMARY

CD SSIs in the United States remain high despite being the focus of recent research. CD SSIs likely have a broader impact on a woman, her newborn, and her family than can be captured by a rate of infections and wound disruption in regard to recovery from the common surgical procedure. There are opportunities for research evaluating rates of depression, prescription opioid abuse, and other quality-of-life measures.

Patient education surrounding postoperative wound care is as important in the prevention of SSI as is adherence to guidelines by surgeons, anesthesia professionals, nurses, and staff.[47] The importance of education on hand hygiene for the patient and her family as well as staff adherence to strict hand washing preoperatively and in the postsurgical period continues to play a major role in prevention of SSI. In addition, patients and family should be educated on early signs and symptoms of wound complications that impact normal wound healing. Staff education programs and refresher courses in aseptic and scrub techniques have been shown to reduce SSI in elective as well as nonelective CD.[20,48]

There is no question that the overall cost of obstetric and postpartum care is impacted by SSI and wound complications following CD. The results of a cost modeling study based on claims data from a single academic tertiary institution found that the direct cost of each case of CD SSI was approximately $3500, although not factoring in indirect costs including costs of outpatient management and lost productivity.[49]

The research also highlights that 1 perioperative change may not have an effective reduction on all SSIs. Each hospital and each region have different patient populations and different challenges. The recent push toward quality improvement projects and bundled interventions can help hospitals find a comprehensive initiative to address SSIs. Instead of relying on 1 new process, a bundle incorporates techniques in an additive fashion. Following a quality improvement process also focuses on standardization and mandates assessment of outcomes.

Optimizing care for women in the postpartum period begins in the preoperative period (**Table 1**). Care after a CD does not end at hospital discharge. Women should be educated on proper wound care following discharge and on the signs and symptoms of early warning of impaired wound healing, such as drainage and pain out of proportion to that expected in the normal healing process. Women should also have follow-up evaluation within the first 3 weeks after CD to evaluate wound healing and any signs that might suggest wound complications.

DISCLOSURE

The author has nothing to disclose.

REFERENCES

1. Yokoe DS, Christiansen CL, Johnson R, et al. Epidemiology of and surveillance for postpartum infections. Emerg Infect Dis 2001;7(5):837–41.

2. Tita ATN, Szychowski JM, Boggess K, et al. Adjunctive azithromycin prophylaxis for cesarean delivery. N Engl J Med 2016;375:1231–41.

3. Villers M, Grotegut C, Edwards J, et al. Factors associated with 30-day readmissions for cesarean delivery surgical site infections. Am J Obstet Gynecol 2016; 215:S819.

4. Skeith AE, Niu B, Valent AM, et al. Adding azithromycin to cephalosporin for cesarean delivery infection prophylaxis: a cost-effectiveness analysis. Obstet Gynecol 2017;130:1279–84.

5. Stamilio DM, Scifres CM. Extreme obesity and postcesarean maternal complications. Obstet Gynecol 2014;124:227–32.

6. Anderson V, Chaboyer W, Gillespie B. The relationship between obesity and surgical site infections in women undergoing caesarean sections: an integrative review. Midwifery 2013;29:1331–8.

7. Pierpont YN, Dinh TP, Salas RE, et al. Obesity and surgical wound healing: a current review. ISRN Obes 2014;2014:638936.

8. Caughey AB, Wood SL, Macones GA, et al. Guidelines for intraoperative care in cesarean delivery: Enhanced Recovery After Surgery Society recommendations (part 2). Am J Obstet Gynecol 2018;219:533–44.

9. Macones GA, Caughey AB, Wood SL, et al. Guidelines for postoperative care in cesarean delivery: Enhanced Recovery After Surgery (ERAS) Society recommendations (part 3). Am J Obstet Gynecol 2019;221:247.e1-.e9.

10. Carter EB, Temming LA, Fowler S, et al. Evidence-based bundles and cesarean delivery surgical site infections: a systematic review and meta-analysis. Obstet Gynecol 2017;130:735–46.

11. Kawakita T, Iqbal SN, Landy HJ, et al. Reducing cesarean delivery surgical site infections: a resident-driven quality initiative. Obstet Gynecol 2019;133:282–8.

12. ACOG Practice Bulletin No. 199 summary: use of prophylactic antibiotics in labor and delivery. Obstet Gynecol 2018;132:798–800.

13. Ahmadzia HK, Patel EM, Joshi D, et al. Obstetric surgical site infections: 2 grams compared with 3 grams of cefazolin in morbidly obese women. Obstet Gynecol 2015;126:708–15.

14. Bourke J, Pavlos R, James I, et al. Improving the effectiveness of penicillin allergy de-labeling. J Allergy Clin Immunol 2015;3:365–74.e1.

15. Moskow JM, Cook N, Champion-Lippmann C, et al. Identifying opportunities in EHR to improve the quality of antibiotic allergy data. J Am Med Inform Assoc 2015;23:e108–12.

16. Harris BS, Hopkins MK, Villers MS, et al. Efficacy of non-beta-lactam antibiotics for prevention of cesarean delivery surgical site infections. AJP Rep 2019;9: e167–71.

17. Tuuli MG, Liu J, Stout MJ, et al. A randomized trial comparing skin antiseptic agents at cesarean delivery. N Engl J Med 2016;374:647–55.

18. Springel EH, Wang X-Y, Sarfoh VM, et al. A randomized open-label controlled trial of chlorhexidine-alcohol vs povidone-iodine for cesarean antisepsis: the CAPICA trial. Am J Obstet Gynecol 2017;217:463.e1-e8.

19. Ngai IM, Van Arsdale A, Govindappagari S, et al. Skin preparation for prevention of surgical site infection after cesarean delivery: a randomized controlled trial. Obstet Gynecol 2015;126:1251–7.

20. Rauk PN. Educational intervention, revised instrument sterilization methods, and comprehensive preoperative skin preparation protocol reduce cesarean section surgical site infections. Am J Infect Control 2010;38:319–23.

21. Caissutti C, Saccone G, Zullo F, et al. Vaginal cleansing before cesarean delivery: a systematic review and meta-analysis. Obstet Gynecol 2017;130:527–38.

22. Haas DM, Morgan S, Contreras K, et al. Vaginal preparation with antiseptic solution before cesarean section for preventing postoperative infections. Cochrane Database Syst Rev 2018;(7):CD007892.

23. Culligan PJ, Kubik K, Murphy M, et al. A randomized trial that compared povidone iodine and chlorhexidine as antiseptics for vaginal hysterectomy. Am J Obstet Gynecol 2005;192:422–5.

24. Boggess KA, Tita A, Jauk V, et al. Risk factors for postcesarean maternal infection in a trial of extended-spectrum antibiotic prophylaxis. Obstet Gynecol 2017;129: 481–5.

25. Alanis MC, Villers MS, Law TL, et al. Complications of cesarean delivery in the massively obese parturient. Am J Obstet Gynecol 2010;203:271.e1-7.

26. Sutton AL, Sanders LB, Subramaniam A, et al. Abdominal incision selection for cesarean delivery of women with class III obesity. Am J Perinatol 2016;33:547–51.

27. Mathai M, Hofmeyr GJ, Mathai NE. Abdominal surgical incisions for caesarean section. Cochrane Database Syst Rev 2013;(5):CD004453.

28. Gizzo S, Andrisani A, Noventa M, et al. Caesarean section: could different transverse abdominal incision techniques influence postpartum pain and subsequent quality of life? A systematic review. PLoS One 2015;10:e0114190.

29. Abalos E, Addo V, Brocklehurst P, et al. Caesarean section surgical techniques: 3 year follow-up of the CORONIS fractional, factorial, unmasked, randomised controlled trial. Lancet 2016;388:62–72.

30. Chelmow D, Rodriguez EJ, Sabatini MM. Suture closure of subcutaneous fat and wound disruption after cesarean delivery: a meta-analysis. Obstet Gynecol 2004; 103:974–80.

31. Berghella V, Baxter JK, Chauhan SP. Evidence-based surgery for cesarean delivery. Am J Obstet Gynecol 2005;193:1607–17.

32. Figueroa D, Jauk VC, Szychowski JM, et al. Surgical staples compared with subcuticular suture for skin closure after cesarean delivery: a randomized controlled trial. Obstet Gynecol 2013;121:33–8.

33. Tuuli MG, Rampersad RM, Carbone JF, et al. Staples compared with subcuticular suture for skin closure after cesarean delivery: a systematic review and meta-analysis. Obstet Gynecol 2011;117:682–90.

34. Mackeen AD, Khalifeh A, Fleisher J, et al. Suture compared with staple skin closure after cesarean delivery: a randomized controlled trial. Obstet Gynecol 2014;123:1169–75.

35. Schrufer-Poland TL, Ruiz MP, Kassar S, et al. Incidence of wound complications in cesarean deliveries following closure with absorbable subcuticular staples versus conventional skin closure techniques. Eur J Obstet Gynecol Reprod Biol 2016;206:53–6.

36. McNulty AK, Schmidt M, Feeley T, et al. Effects of negative pressure wound therapy on fibroblast viability, chemotactic signaling, and proliferation in a provisional wound (fibrin) matrix. Wound Repair Regen 2007;15:838–46.

37. Echebiri NC, McDoom MM, Aalto MM, et al. Prophylactic use of negative pressure wound therapy after cesarean delivery. Obstet Gynecol 2015;125:299–307.

38. Yu L, Kronen RJ, Simon LE, et al. Prophylactic negative-pressure wound therapy after cesarean is associated with reduced risk of surgical site infection: a systematic review and meta-analysis. Am J Obstet Gynecol 2018;218:200–10.e1.

39. Hyldig N, Vinter CA, Kruse M, et al. Prophylactic incisional negative pressure wound therapy reduces the risk of surgical site infection after caesarean section in obese women: a pragmatic randomised clinical trial. BJOG 2019;126:628–35.
40. Paz Maya S, Dualde Beltran D, Lemercier P, et al. Necrotizing fasciitis: an urgent diagnosis. Skeletal Radiol 2014;43:577–89.
41. Sama CB, Tankou CS, Angwafo Iii FF. Fulminating postcaesarean necrotising fasciitis: a rare and lethal condition successfully managed in a resource-disadvantaged setting in sub-Saharan Africa. Case Rep Obstet Gynecol 2017; 2017:9763470.
42. Hakkarainen TW, Kopari NM, Pham TN, et al. Necrotizing soft tissue infections: review and current concepts in treatment, systems of care, and outcomes. Curr Probl Surg 2014;51:344–62.
43. Falola RA, Ward CM, Kim MJ, et al. Potential future applications for negative pressure wound therapy and installation devices. Surg Technol Int 2016;30:55–60.
44. Dodson MK, Magann EF, Gr Meeks. A randomized comparison of secondary closure and secondary intention in patients with superficial wound dehiscence. Obstet Gynecol 1992;80(3):321–4.
45. Wechter ME, Pearlman MD, Hartmann KE. Reclosure of the disrupted laparotomy wound: a systematic review. Obstet Gynecol 2005;106:376–83.
46. Tilt A, Falola RA, Kumar A, et al. Operative management of abdominal wound dehiscence: outcomes and factors influencing time to healing in patients undergoing surgical debridement with primary closure. Wounds 2018;30:317–23.
47. Tartari E, Weterings V, Gastmeier P, et al. Patient engagement with surgical site infection prevention: an expert panel perspective. Antimicrob Resist Infect Control 2017;6:45.
48. Zuarez-Easton S, Zafran N, Garmi G, et al. Postcesarean wound infection: prevalence, impact, prevention, and management challenges. Int J Womens Health 2017;9:81–8.
49. Olsen MA, Butler AM, Willers DM, et al. Comparison of costs of surgical site infection and endometritis after cesarean section using claims and medical record data. Infect Control Hosp Epidemiol 2010;31(8):872–5.

Stillbirth
Evaluation and Follow-up

Jessica M. Page, M.D., Robert M. Silver, MD*

KEYWORDS

- Stillbirth • Evaluation • Cause of death • Postpartum

KEY POINTS

- The highest-yield diagnostic tests following a stillbirth are fetal autopsy, placental pathology, and genetic testing.
- Diagnostic testing following a stillbirth should be tailored to the clinical scenario, and patients should be given timely, accurate information regarding their options and expected yield of each test.
- Grief following stillbirth is experienced in different ways, and providers should ensure patients have access to appropriate support services.
- Identifying a cause of death facilitates emotional healing and closure for patients and informs recurrence risk and future pregnancy management.

INTRODUCTION

Stillbirth is defined in the United States as fetal death at 20 weeks' gestation and greater. In the United States, the rate of stillbirth exceeds that of other high-income countries at 5.96 per 1000 births with an annual rate reduction that lags behind that of many high-income countries.[1,2] In order to improve this, better identification of causes of fetal death is needed so that prevention strategies may be developed. In real-world practice, up to two-thirds of stillbirths are unexplained.[3,4] The proportion of unexplained stillbirths can be reduced with a systematic, thorough approach to stillbirth evaluation. In a large prospective cohort of stillbirth cases, only 24% were left unexplained following a uniform, thorough evaluation.[5] This finding highlights the need for improved stillbirth care in the United States, which can be achieved in part by educating patients and providers on the options and yield of various diagnostic tests following a stillbirth.

Evaluation

Identifying a potential cause of death after a stillbirth is important for both families and providers. For patients, this process can help to facilitate bereavement, healing, and

Department of Obstetrics and Gynecology, University of Utah Health, 30 North 1900 East, Suite 2A200, Salt Lake City, UT 84132, USA
* Corresponding author.
E-mail address: Bob.silver@hsc.utah.edu

Obstet Gynecol Clin N Am 47 (2020) 439–451
https://doi.org/10.1016/j.ogc.2020.04.008
0889-8545/20/© 2020 Elsevier Inc. All rights reserved.

obgyn.theclinics.com

emotional closure. It is also an integral step in determining the likelihood of a recurrent stillbirth and identifying areas for preventive strategies in future pregnancies. The provision of accurate, thorough information regarding the evaluation of stillbirth in a sensitive and timely manner from trusted health care providers is crucial. In the wake of this devastating event, it is often difficult for families to navigate this decision-making process, particularly when it comes to making choices regarding fetal autopsy and genetic testing. It is common for families to think that this testing will not bring back their baby or change the situation. Concerns regarding cost also create barriers that can often be addressed with accurate information and targeted testing. However, families often have regrets when they do not perform an evaluation for causes of stillbirth, and failure to perform a "workup" makes counseling and management of subsequent pregnancies difficult. Thus, it is important for providers to be knowledgeable and prepared to counsel families regarding both the options and the yield of each component of a stillbirth evaluation.

Defining a cause of death following a stillbirth can be difficult due in part to the fact that a stillbirth can be caused by a multitude of conditions and that clinical clues are often lacking. In addition, there are many different classification systems for determining a cause of stillbirth.[6] These systems use varying components of the clinical history, laboratory results, and pathologic examination results to identify a potential cause of death or contributing conditions to fetal death. The yield and accuracy of these systems vary based on the setting and information available. For example, some systems are designed for use in middle- and low-income countries and thus do not include many technologically advanced and expensive tests owing to limited resources.[6,7] This likely results in less accurate causes of death and a higher proportion of unexplained cases as compared with a high-income setting with numerous resources for evaluation. In high-resource settings, a thorough evaluation of stillbirth leads to identification of a probable or possible cause of death in 76% of cases.[5]

Historically, many tests have been performed following a stillbirth, but with varying yields on the ultimate determination of a cause of death. Given the often unclear and heterogeneous circumstances surrounding a stillbirth, it is important to use the most effective tests for the clinical scenario. Unfortunately, it has been shown that up to two-thirds of stillbirth cases remain unexplained, highlighting the need for a consistent, effective evaluation approach.[3,4] The American College of Obstetricians and Gynecologists currently recommends an extensive approach to stillbirth evaluation.[8] This approach includes a thorough clinical history as well as an array of tests. The utility of common stillbirth evaluation tests in identifying or ruling out a cause of death was determined in a secondary analysis of a large US stillbirth cohort. An approach to stillbirth evaluation based on the clinical scenario was provided and is shown in **Fig. 1**.[9]

Maternal Medical and Pregnancy History

A detailed medical and pregnancy history is of utmost importance in determining a potential cause of death in a stillbirth case. This evaluation begins with a detailed history and physical examination. Attention should be paid to preexisting maternal medical conditions, such as chronic hypertension, diabetes, autoimmune diseases, and other. The family history can also be useful if relatives have had pregnancies complicated by stillbirth, recurrent early pregnancy loss, fetal malformations, or genetic abnormalities.

The clinical scenario leading up to the presentation with stillbirth can also be extremely informative. Pregnancy complications, such as known fetal anomalies, fetal

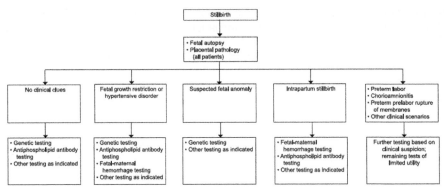

Fig. 1. Suggested stillbirth evaluation test recommendations based on the clinical scenario. (*From* Page JM, Christiansen-Lindquist L, Thorsten V, et al. Diagnostic tests for evaluation of stillbirth: results from the stillbirth collaborative research network. Obstet Gynecol 2017;129(4):705; with permission.)

growth abnormalities, hypertensive disorders of pregnancy, multifetal gestation, or a preterm labor process, can point to a pathophysiologic pathway leading to fetal death. In addition, symptoms and signs, such as vaginal bleeding, abdominal pain, fever, sweats, chills, provide clues for potential causes, such as abruption, fetal-maternal hemorrhage, preterm labor, and various infections.

Fetal Autopsy

A detailed postmortem examination or fetal autopsy is one of the most important components of a stillbirth evaluation. It has had a very high clinical yield in finding a potential cause of death in several studies. A large prospectively collected cohort of stillbirth cases in the United States found that fetal autopsy was helpful in determining a cause of death in 42% of cases.[9] Usefulness was determined as a positive finding that confirmed a suspected cause of death or a negative finding that excluded a cause of death.[9] Using similar definitions, a large prospective Dutch stillbirth cohort found fetal autopsy to be valuable for identification of a cause of death in 73% of cases. This cohort used a different classification system and was restricted to antepartum stillbirths, perhaps explaining the different percentages.[10] An additional US study evaluated the major components of stillbirth workup to assess the stepwise contribution of each component to finding a cause of death. This investigation found that fetal autopsy, when added to clinical and laboratory information as well as placental pathology, increased diagnostic yield for a cause of death from 61% to 74% of cases. Not all studies have had such favorable results for fetal autopsy. For example, 1 group noted only a 1% to 2% improvement in the identification of a cause of death when autopsy was added to placental pathology and clinical data.[11] In this study, approximately 60% of stillbirths remained unexplained. Again, the use of different classification systems, which place varied emphasis on individual components of the evaluation, may account for discrepant findings among studies.

The quality and yield of fetal autopsy depend on the availability of specialized perinatal pathologists. These individuals have specific training in fetal and placental examinations and are of utmost importance to the diagnostic evaluation following a stillbirth. As a provider, it is important to familiarize oneself with the policies and procedures for fetal autopsy at local facilities, and if needed, identify the closest referral center with a perinatal pathologist. The time interval from delivery to pathologic examination does not have a significant impact on examination yield. Thus, in some situations, transport of the child for examination by a perinatal pathologist may be appropriate.[11]

Fetal autopsy is remarkably underused in many centers. For example, a study of fetal death certificate data between 2010 and 2014 in 2 US centers revealed that fetal autopsy is completed in only 12% to 24% of cases and that this rate is declining.[12] Patient barriers to completion of fetal autopsy include concerns regarding invasiveness of the procedure, timing and transport, organ retention issues, emotional distress, and poor understanding of the value of the procedure.[13] There also may be cultural or religious concerns about autopsies and misconceptions regarding the procedure. Providers also contribute to a low completion rate because of feelings of lack of qualification to discuss autopsy. Also, they fear that the discussion may increase stress for the family, and they may want to avoid an uncomfortable conversation.[14] Moreover, knowledge regarding options for a less-invasive examination or alternatives, such as MRI, may increase utilization.[15] Given the above perceived barriers, it is important for providers to become familiar with the logistics of fetal autopsy in their institutions and to clearly communicate the importance of this examination to determining a cause of death to patients. The benefits of identifying a cause of death should be emphasized, including emotional closure and improved ability to predict recurrence risk and targeted risk reduction in future pregnancies. A survey of patients following stillbirth revealed that most patients did not complete fetal autopsy because of concern regarding cost and lack of utility.[16] The utility and logistics of fetal autopsy are clear targets for education because in many institutions autopsy is free to families and is one of the highest-yield examinations in a stillbirth workup.[9,10] Also, families often regret not performing a fetal autopsy, and provider counseling has a major impact on decision making.[17]

Placental Pathology

Placental pathology is one of the highest-yield components of a stillbirth evaluation and is widely available and acceptable. The quality of this examination, like fetal autopsy, is influenced by access to a perinatal pathologist. Also, it is performed more often with easy availability. Pathologic placental changes are implicated in 23% to 65% of stillbirths in large cohort studies.[5,10,11,15] Given this, placental pathology has high yield in identifying a potential cause of death. In a large US cohort study, placental pathology helped to identify or rule out a suspected cause of death in 65% of stillbirth cases.[9] It was useful in every clinical scenario, including those without clinical clues suggestive of a potential cause of death.[9] Similarly, in a Dutch stillbirth cohort, placental pathology was helpful in 96% of cases.[10] When analyzed in a stepwise fashion, addition of placental pathology to clinical and laboratory information increased diagnostic yield from 24% to 61%.[18] This striking utility emphasizes the importance of assessing placental pathology following all stillbirth cases.

Genetic Testing

Genetic testing can provide important information regarding the pathophysiologic process leading to stillbirth. Genetic abnormalities have been implicated in 6% to 17% of stillbirths with higher rates in those complicated by fetal anomalies.[19-21] Technologies for genetic testing include karyotype, chromosomal microarray, and evolving new techniques, such as whole-genome or whole-exome sequencing. Testing has been traditionally performed with karyotype analysis. However, this had limited yield because it requires live cells to grow and divide in culture, which are not always available after stillbirth. In a large series of US stillbirth cases, chromosomal microarray increased the diagnostic yield from 71% to 87% because it can detect smaller copy number changes and does not rely on live tissue.[22] Given the widespread availability of this test and relative affordability, it is the recommended genetic evaluation following stillbirth in most cases.[8] Whole-exome sequencing and whole-genome sequencing provide the highest-resolution genetic technology available and are increasingly used in clinical genetic diagnosis. Whole-exome sequencing increases the prenatal detection of pathogenic variants in anomalous fetuses by 8% to 24%.[23,24] Whole-exome sequencing and whole-genome sequencing have not been extensively studied in stillbirth cases to date and have been reserved for select cases, such as those affected by unexplained nonimmune hydrops.[25,26] The types of genetic abnormalities observed in stillbirths are similar to live births; the most frequent are monosomy X, trisomy 21, trisomy 18, trisomy 13 as well as mosaics, autosomal monosomies, deletions, and unbalanced translocations.[21]

Infection

In high-income countries, approximately 10% to 20% of stillbirths are due to infection.[5,27] Infection leads to fetal death through several pathophysiologic pathways, including direct fetal infection, placental infection leading to placental insufficiency, severe maternal illness, and infection involved in previable or periviable preterm birth. Assigning a cause of death to infection is complex because isolated serologic, culture, or histopathologic evidence of infection alone cannot assign causality if not supported by the clinical scenario. Most infection-related stillbirths are multifactorial. A secondary analysis of infection-related stillbirth cases showed that 32% had infection as a sole cause of death, and 68% had multiple causes present. In the multifactorial cases, the most common additional causes included spontaneous preterm delivery (69%) and placental causes (24%).[28] The predominant pathogens identified in infection-related stillbirths in high-resource settings are *Escherichia coli* (29%), group B streptococcus (12%), and enterococcus (12%), which speak to the predominance of preterm birth pathophysiology in this population.[28]

Testing for specific organisms, such as parvovirus and syphilis, has been recommended.[8] Parvovirus is implicated in stillbirth because it can destroy fetal erythroid progenitor cells, leading to severe fetal anemia, hydrops, and cardiovascular failure.[29] It also may directly affect the fetal heart, leading to hydrops. However, most cases of acute maternal parvovirus infection during pregnancy are asymptomatic and result in the birth of a healthy infant. Accordingly, a positive maternal serologic test for parvovirus without corresponding clinical evidence of fetal parvovirus infection with elevated middle cerebral artery Doppler, hydrops, or findings on fetal autopsy or placental pathology indicates that parvovirus is very unlikely to be the cause of death. In fact, in the SCRN study, out of 55 patients tested for parvovirus immunoglobulin M (IgM) antibodies, 5 had a positive result, indicating acute infection. However, this was the suspected cause of death in only 2 of these cases because they also had corresponding clinical and histologic evidence of fetal parvovirus infection.[28] Thus, testing for parvovirus should be guided by the clinical scenario because it is not useful as a screening test in an otherwise unexplained stillbirth case. The pathogenic organism in syphilis is the spirochete *Treponema pallidum*. The prevalence in high-income areas is as low as 0.02%, but in endemic low-income areas, it can be as high as 20%.[27] In the United States, the prevalence of syphilis was 9.5 cases per 100,000 people in 2017, which was a 73% increase since 2013 with a corresponding increase in the number of congenital syphilis cases.[30] Syphilis can cause infection in the placenta and fetus and most often results in fetal death through placental inflammation and insufficiency.[31] If untreated, syphilis can result in fetal death in approximately 40%

of cases.[27] These factors underscore the importance of screening for and treating syphilis in pregnancy. In an analysis of 66 infection-related stillbirths in the United States, syphilis was the causative organism in 1 case (1.5%) in which spirochetes were noted on placental pathology and fetal autopsy in the setting of a positive serologic screening result.[28] Testing for syphilis should be performed if no screen has yet been performed in pregnancy, if the patient has risk factors for sexually transmitted disease exposure, or if findings indicative of syphilis infection are noted on fetal autopsy or placental pathology. In low-income countries, up to 50% of stillbirth cases are attributable to infection.[27] The high rate of infectionrelated stillbirth is due in large part to a higher prevalence of malaria and syphilis, both of which can cause fetal death by placental infection resulting in insufficiency or direct fetal infection.[27]

There are limited data to support routine testing for other "TORCH" (toxoplasmosis, rubella, cytomegalovirus [CMV], and herpes virus) organisms.[8] Of these, CMV is the most common congenital infection and has been the most frequently noted TORCH organism in an assessment of infection-related stillbirth.[27,28] Of the cases in which CMV infection was the suspected cause of death (5 of 66 cases, 7.6%), viral inclusion bodies were noted on placental pathology or fetal autopsy. Because many fetuses born to mothers with acute CMV infection have no adverse sequelae, these histologic findings are much stronger indicators of pathogenic infection compared with maternal serology.[28] Similar findings were noted for herpes simplex virus (HSV) with 1 case (1.5%) having positive placental or fetal histologic findings.[28] Toxoplasmosis and rubella are exceedingly rare causes of stillbirth in the United States. Thus, screening is of questionable benefit unless infection is suggested by the clinical scenario or by histopathology.

Fetal and placental cultures have also been used in the evaluation of infection in stillbirth cases. These methods have variable yield and accuracy. They are best performed at the time of pathologic examination of the fetus and placenta. A targeted evaluation for infection-related stillbirth is included in **Fig. 2.**

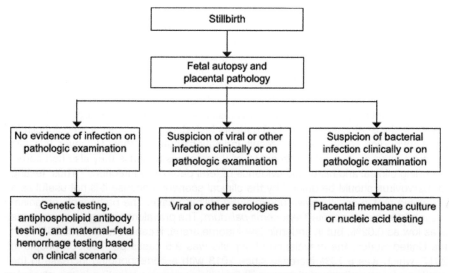

Fig. 2. Depicting the work-up of a suspected infection-related stillbirth. (*From* Page JM, Bardsley T, Thorsten V, et al. Stillbirth Associated With Infection in a Diverse U.S. Cohort. Obstet Gynecol 2019;134(6):1195; with permission.)

Laboratory Tests

Antiphospholipid syndrome (APS) is a condition that is diagnosed according to clinical criteria with confirmatory laboratory testing. Clinical criteria for APS include venous, arterial, or small-vessel thrombosis as well as pregnancy complications, including fetal death (>10 weeks' gestation), severe preeclampsia or placental insufficiency requiring delivery before 34 weeks, or 3 or more pregnancy losses before 10 weeks' gestation.[32] Laboratory testing for APS involves maternal testing for lupus anticoagulant, anti-β-2-glycoprotein-I IgG/IgM antibodies, and anticardiolipin IgG/IgM antibodies. A positive test occurs with a positive screen for lupus anticoagulant (LA) or with elevated levels of antibodies greater than the 99th percentile on 2 occasions performed 12 weeks apart.[32] A large stillbirth case-control study found that elevated levels of anticardiolipin IgG and anti-β-2-glycoprotein-I IgG were associated with a 3-fold increase in the risk of stillbirth (odds ratio [OR]: 3.43; 95% confidence interval [CI]: 1.79-6.60). This association of elevated anticardiolipin IgG antibodies with stillbirth was more pronounced when excluding stillbirths complicated by fetal anomalies or obstetric complications (OR: 5.30; 95% CI: 2.39-11.76).[33] In a secondary analysis of this cohort, testing for antiphospholipid antibodies was useful in identifying or ruling out a cause of death in 11% of cases. This utility was increased to 28% to 32% in cases complicated by fetal growth restriction or hypertensive disorders of pregnancy.[9]

Fetal-maternal hemorrhage is implicated in the pathophysiologic process leading to stillbirth in 1% to 13% of cases.[34,35] Severe fetal anemia leads to fetal compromise, and the risk is highest with hemorrhage of 20 mL/kg or more.[35] Evaluation for fetal-maternal hemorrhage is a time-sensitive test given that assesses the level of fetal hemoglobin present in the maternal circulation. It is ideally performed at the time of presentation with a fetal death because it can be elevated by delivery itself. However, in the case of large hemorrhages, testing may be positive up to 3 weeks after delivery. Testing can be accomplished with a Kleihauer-Betke test or flow cytometry. The Kleihauer-Betke test may result in an underestimation of fetal-maternal hemorrhage because it only assesses a small number of cells.[36] In a US prospective stillbirth cohort, 43.6% of cases were tested for fetal-maternal hemorrhage, and 4.6% of them had a positive test.[5] In this cohort, testing for fetal-maternal hemorrhage was considered useful in 6.4% of cases.[9] In a Dutch prospective stillbirth cohort, 12% of cases were positive for fetal-maternal hemorrhage, and it was considered a cause of death in only 1.3% of cases.[10] Given the narrow window for testing and relative utility, testing for fetal-maternal hemorrhage is recommended in otherwise unexplained stillbirths.[9]

Testing for other maternal medical complications should be driven by clues from the clinical presentation. Relevant conditions include but are not limited to diabetes and systemic lupus erythematosus (SLE). In the setting of a large-for-gestational-age fetus, it may be reasonable to test for diabetes. Similarly, if clinical manifestations of lupus are present, assessment for SLE is warranted. However, testing for subclinical diabetes, thyroid disease, or other medical conditions is not recommended based on existing data. Rare conditions contributing to stillbirth, such as illicit drug use or intrahepatic of cholestasis of pregnancy, should be assessed if suspected based on the clinical presentation, but otherwise are not part of recommended screening.[37] Historically, testing for inherited thrombophilias was suggested as part of routine stillbirth evaluation. However, large studies have shown that the association between thrombophilias and stillbirth is weak and that treatment does not show clear benefit.[38,39]

The Postpartum Visit

Given the emotional stress following stillbirth, early and perhaps several postpartum visits are warranted. Following stillbirth, patients have reported the need for a clear postpartum follow-up plan before leaving the hospital, which should ideally be made with the primary obstetric provider.[40] Goals of this visit are to address emotional healing and the support system for the patient and her family, the stillbirth evaluation and results leading to a potential cause of death, as well as recurrence risk and future pregnancy management if desired.

Healing after a stillbirth involves acknowledgment and validation of the families' grief, addressing the child that was lost, and a careful review of the pregnancy and events leading up to the fetal death. A dual-process model of grief, rather than a linear model, has been proposed to be more applicable to emotional recovery after stillbirth.[41] In this model, persons alternate between 2 modes, the "loss orientation mode" and the "restoration orientation mode." These modes are described in **Table 1**. This model addresses the fact that grief is an individual process that is experienced differently by each person. This framework is helpful for providers to try and meet patients and their families "where they are" in each of their grief processes. It is also important to address evolving psychiatric disorders as a patient recovers following a stillbirth. There is a high risk of progression to depression and anxiety, particularly in the first year following a stillbirth.[42]

In addition, it is important to continually validate the families' loss, use the child's name, and review the events leading to the death. Following stillbirth, 52% of patients reported having a poor understanding of the events surround the stillbirth, and 71% were dissatisfied with the information they received,[41] highlighting the importance of using the postpartum visits to review the clinical course and results of the evaluation. It may also be an opportunity to complete portions of the evaluation that were not done at the time of diagnosis or delivery. Depending on the interval from delivery, fetal autopsy and placental pathology may still be feasible, as are many of the laboratory tests described above. Surveys of parents experiencing stillbirth have found that they value

Table 1	
The dual-process model of grief	
Loss Orientation	**Restoration Orientation**
Confrontation of the loss	Adjustment to the loss
Talking	Evading
"Being"	"Doing"
Denial and avoidance of recovery	Denial and avoidance of loss
Involvement	Distance
Closeness	Aloofness
Need for emotional support	Need to problem-solve
"Chronic mourning"	"Postponed mourning"
Dangers: complaining, overinvolvement, drowning in emotion	Dangers: escapism, distance, overcontrol, feeling nothing

From Heazell AE, Leisher S, Cregan M, et al. Sharing experiences to improve bereavement support and clinical care after stillbirth: report of the 7th annual meeting of the International Stillbirth Alliance. Acta Obstet Gynecol Scand 2013;92(3):353; with permission.

honesty and directness from providers, and they urged obstetric caregivers to act as informed guides in the process of navigating the complex decisions around stillbirth evaluation.[41] Providers can also offer resources for support outside the health care setting. Resources for support can be particularly helpful because patients can connect with individuals who have experienced similar losses, learn of advocacy opportunities and other ways to help them with their healing process. There are organizations in the United States with online resources and contact information (https://www.cdc.gov/ncbddd/stillbirth/resources.html).

Caring for patients and families experiencing a stillbirth can also be emotionally taxing for providers. There are limited data on providers' experience with stillbirth care, but it is an important area in need of further attention. In 1 study, 1 in 10 providers reported considering stopping obstetric practice because of the emotional stress of caring for a patient with stillbirth.[43] This finding highlights the importance of developing peer and family relationships for emotional support during and after these experiences and seeking additional health care as needed. Internationally, modules have been developed to assist health care providers in addressing family care, physical care, psychosocial care, cultural care, and self-care following a perinatal loss.[41] Such a formalized program does not exist in the United States and is a target for advancement in health care locally.

Counseling following a stillbirth also involves addressing the results of the evaluation, potential causes of death, and recurrence risk. As discussed above, the task of assigning a cause of death is complex, and many different classification systems exist.[6] It is reasonable for care providers to synthesize the clinical data and either familiarize oneself with a commonly used classification system or discuss the case with a maternal-fetal medicine specialist or other person with experience in perinatal cause of death audits. At some institutions, there are groups of providers who will provide a review of a stillbirth case and provide a potential cause of death, personalized recurrence risk estimates, and management strategies for future pregnancies.

In general, without taking gestational age or cause of death into account, a patient who has had 1 stillbirth is 6 times (hazard ratio [HR]: 5.8; 95% CI: 3.7–9.0) more likely to experience a recurrent fetal loss as compared with a patient with a prior live birth.[44] Similar studies have found a 2- to 10-fold increased risk of recurrent stillbirth as compared with individuals with prior live birth.[45–47] The highest risk for recurrent loss follows stillbirths at 20 to 23 weeks (relative risk [RR]: 2.81; 95% CI: 1.4–5.6), 28 to 31 weeks (RR: 2.6; 95% CI: 1.1–6.1), and 40 weeks and above (RR: 3.5; 95% CI: 1.4–8.7).[48]

Addressing management of future pregnancies is an important component of postpartum care following a stillbirth. In 1 study, 66% of women conceived within a year of a stillbirth, highlighting the need for an organized plan of care during the postpartum period.[49] A large, international retrospective cohort study evaluated the effect of interpregnancy interval following a stillbirth and subsequent pregnancy outcomes. Women conceiving within 12 months did not have an increased risk of adverse pregnancy outcomes compared with women waiting 24 to 59 months.[50] Thus, it is reasonable to support patients to pursue a subsequent pregnancy when they are emotionally and physically ready.

Recurrent stillbirth risk-reduction strategies include addressing modifiable risk factors, antenatal surveillance, and delivery planning. Risk factors that should be addressed, ideally beginning as early as the postpartum visit, include smoking cessation, discontinuation of any illicit drug use, and weight loss. Given the increased stillbirth risk associated with multiple gestations, care should be taken with assisted reproduction technologies. Optimization of ongoing maternal medical issues, such as diabetes, chronic hypertension, and SLE, should also be achieved.[51]

Medical interventions have also been proposed with a goal of improving placental function. Low-dose aspirin has been evaluated in a large metaanalysis, and a 14% reduction in fetal or neonatal death was found. This reduction in fetal or neonatal death may have been due to reduction in preeclampsia, preterm birth, and fetal growth restriction; thus, these data should be interpreted with caution.[52] At this time, routine use of low-dose aspirin is not indicated for history of stillbirth without other risk factors for preeclampsia.[53] Low-molecular-weight heparin as well as prednisolone and hydroxychloroquine hasnot been shown to be consistently effective in preventing pregnancy loss, and data regarding their use outside of SLE or APS are lacking.[51,54,55]

Antenatal surveillance strategies include nonstress tests (NSTs), biophysical profiles (BPPs), and fetal movement assessments. These tests are based on the assumption that the fetal heart pattern and physical activity are affected by fetal hypoxia and acidemia.[56] The risk of fetal death following a reactive NST is about 1.9 per 1000 births,[57] and the risk of fetal death following a normal BPP (score 8 or 10) or modified BPP (NST and amniotic fluid index) is approximately 0.8 per 1000 births.[57–59] There are no clear guidelines that dictate how best to use these tests in subsequent pregnancies following a stillbirth. Antenatal testing must be done with the acknowledgment of the risk for false positive results and thus potentially unnecessary iatrogenic preterm or early term delivery. To balance this risk with that of potential fetal compromise, it is reasonable to initiate antenatal surveillance at 32 to 34 weeks' gestation.[8] If other maternal or pregnancy-related comorbidities are present, such as chronic hypertension, diabetes, or monochorionic multiple gestation, the initiation of testing should be dictated by those conditions.

Early delivery is an attractive strategy for stillbirth risk reduction, but this must be balanced with the risks of prematurity. The risk of infant mortality owing to late preterm birth is 8.8 per 1000 births at 32 to 33 weeks' gestation and 3 per 1000 births at 34 to 36 weeks' gestation.[60] Currently, delivery at 39 weeks' gestation is recommended unless indicated earlier because of abnormal testing or other maternal or pregnancy-related comorbidities.[60]

SUMMARY

Care following a stillbirth is centered on providing accurate information regarding options for evaluation, a careful review of the clinical circumstances, and ongoing follow-up of the patient's emotional healing as well as management of future pregnancies. The highest-yield diagnostic tests include fetal autopsy, placental pathology, and genetic testing in addition to a thorough clinical history.[9,10] These tests should be offered to all patients after a stillbirth. A test for fetal-maternal hemorrhage is also recommended given the time-sensitive nature of this evaluation. Further testing should be informed according to the clinical setting.[9] Identification of a potential cause of death can provide emotional closure for families and inform recurrence risk as well as management of future pregnancies.

DISCLOSURE

The authors have nothing to disclose.

REFERENCES

1. MacDorman MF, Gregory EC. Fetal and perinatal mortality: United States, 2013. Natl Vital Stat Rep 2015;64:1–24.

2. Flenady V, Wojcieszek AM, Middleton P, et al. Stillbirths: recall to action in high-income countries. Lancet 2016;387:691–702.
3. Fretts RC. Etiology and prevention of stillbirth. Am J Obstet Gynecol 2005;193: 1923–35.
4. Goldenberg RL, Kirby R, Culhane JF. Stillbirth: a review. J Matern Fetal Neonatal Med 2004;16:79–94.
5. Stillbirth Collaborative Research Network Writing Group. Causes of death among stillbirths. JAMA 2011;306:2459–68.
6. Flenady V, Wojcieszek AM, Ellwood D. Classification of causes and associated conditions for stillbirths and neonatal deaths. Semin Fetal Neonat Med 2017; 22:176–85.
7. Leisher SH, Teoh Z, Reinebrant H, et al. Classification systems for causes of still-birth and neonatal death, 2009-2014: an assessment of alignment with character-istics for an effective global system. BMC Pregnancy Childbirth 2016;16:269.
8. Management of stillbirth. ACOG Practice Bulletin No. 102. American College of Obstetricians and Gynecologists. Obstet Gynecol 2009;113:748–61.
9. Page JM, Christiansen-Lindquist L, Thorsten V, et al. Diagnostic tests for evalua-tion of stillbirth: results from the Stillbirth Collaborative Research Network. Obstet Gynecol 2017;129:699–706.
10. Korteweg FJ, Eerwich JJ, Timmer A, et al. Evaluation of 1025 fetal deaths: pro-posed diagnostic workup. Am J Obstet Gynecol 2012;206:53.e1-2.
11. Man J, Hutchinson JC, Heazell AE, et al. Stillbirth and intrauterine fetal death: fac-tors affecting determination of cause of death at autopsy. Ultrasound Obstet Gy-necol 2016;48:566–73.
12. Forsberg K, Christiansen-Lindquist L, Silver RM. Factors associated with stillbirth autopsy in Georgia and Utah, 2010-2014: the importance of delivery location. Am J Perinatol 2018;35(13):1271–80.
13. Lewis C, Hill M, Arthurs OJ, et al. Factors affecting uptake of postmortem exam-ination in the prenatal, perinatal and paediatric setting. BJOG 2017. https://doi.org/10.1111/1471-0528.14600.
14. Heazell AE, McLaughlin MJ, Schmidt EB, et al. A difficult conversation? The views and experiences of parents and professionals on the consent process for peri-natal postmortem after stillbirth. BJOG 2012;119:987–97.
15. McPherson E, Nestoridi E, Heinke D, et al. Alternatives to autopsy for fetal and early neonatal (perinatal) deaths: insights from the Wisconsin Stillbirth Service Program. Birth Defects Res 2017;109(18):1430–41.
16. Warland J, O'Brien LM, Heazell AE, et al. An international internet survey of the experiences of 1,714 mothers with a late stillbirth: the STARS cohort study. BMC Pregnancy Childbirth 2015;15:172.
17. Rankin J, Wright C, Lind T. Cross sectional survey of parents' experience and views of the postmortem examination. BMJ 2002;324(7341):816–8.
18. Miller ES, Minturn L, Linn R, et al. Stillbirth evaluation: a stepwise assessment of placental pathology and autopsy. Am J Obstet Gynecol 2016;214:115.e1-6.
19. Christiaens GC, Vissers J, Poddighe PJ, et al. Comparative genomic hybridiza-tion for cytogenetic evaluation of stillbirth. Obstet Gynecol 2000;96:281–6.
20. Korteweg FJ, Bouman K, Erwich JJ, et al. Cytogenetic analysis after evaluation of 750 fetal deaths: proposal from diagnostic workup. Obstet Gynecol 2008;111: 865–74.
21. Wapner RJ. Genetics of stillbirth. Clin Obstet Gynecol 2010;53(3):628–34.
22. Reddy UM, Page GP, Saade GR, et al. Karyotype versus microarray testing for genetic abnormalities after stillbirth. N Engl J Med 2012;367:2185–93.

23. Fu F, Li R, Li Y. Whole exome sequencing as a diagnostic adjunct to clinical testing in fetuses with structural abnormalities. Ultrasound Obstet Gynecol 2018;51(4):493–502.

24. Lord J, McMullan DJ, Eberhardt RY, et al, Prenatal Assessment of Genomes and Exomes Consortium. Prenatal exome sequencing analysis in fetal structural anomalies detected by ultrasonography (PAGE): a cohort study. Lancet 2019; 393(10173):747–57.

25. Shamseldin HE, Kurdi W, Almusafri F, et al. Molecular autopsy in maternal-fetal medicine. Genet Med 2018;20(4):420–7.

26. Yates CL, Monaghan KG, Copenheaver D, et al. Whole-exome sequencing on deceased fetuses with ultrasound anomalies: expanding our knowledge of genetic disease during fetal development. Genet Med 2017;19(10):1171–8.

27. Goldenberg RL, McClure EM, Saleem S, et al. Infection-related stillbirths. Lancet 2010;375:1482–90.

28. Page JM, Bardsley T, Thorsten V, et al. Stillbirth associated with infection in a diverse U.S. cohort. Obstet Gynecol 2019;134(6):1187–96.

29. Anderson LJ, Hurwitz ES. Human parvovirus B19 and pregnancy. Clin Perinatol 1988;15:273–86.

30. Centers for Disease Control and Prevention. National profile overview-syphilis. USA: Sexually Transmitted Disease Surveillance, Atlanta, Georgia; 2017. Available at: https://www.cdc.gov/std/stats17/syphilis.htm.

31. Sheffield JS, Sanchez PJ, Wendel GD, et al. Placental histopathology of congenital syphilis. Obstet Gynecol 2002;100:126–33.

32. Miyakis S, Lockshin MD, Atsumi T, et al. International consensus statement on an update of the classification criteria for definite antiphospholipid syndrome (APS). J Thromb Haemost 2006;4:295–306.

33. Silver RM, Parker CB, Reddy UM, et al. Antiphospholipid antibodies in stillbirth. Obstet Gynecol 2013;122:641–57.

34. Laube DW, Schauberger CW. Fetomaternal bleeding as a cause for 'unexplained' fetal death. Obstet Gynecol 1982;60:649–51.

35. Rubod C, Deruelle P, Le Goueff F, et al. Long-term prognosis for infants after massive fetomaternal hemorrhage. Obstet Gynecol 2007;110(2 Pt 1):256–60.

36. Sebring ES, Polesky HF. Fetomaternal hemorrhage: incidence, risk factors, time of occurrence, and clinical effects. Transfusion 1990;30:344–51.

37. Silver RM, Parker CB, Goldenberg R, et al. Bile acids in a multicenter, population-based case-control study of stillbirth. Am J Obstet Gynecol 2014; 210:460.e1-9.

38. Rodger MA, Hague WM, Kingdom J, et al. Antepartum dalteparin versus no antepartum dalteparin for the prevention of pregnancy complications in pregnant women with thrombophilia (TIPPS): a multinational open-label randomized trial. Lancet 2014;384:1673–83.

39. Silver RM, Saade GR, Thorsten V, et al. Factor V Leiden, prothrombin G20210A, and methylene tetrahydrofolate reductase mutations and stillbirth: the stillbirth collaborative research network. Am J Obstet Gynecol 2016;215:468.e1-17.

40. Siassakos D, Jackson S, Gleeson K, et al. All bereaved parents are entitled to good care after stillbirth: a mixed-methods multicentre study (INSIGHT). BJOG 2018;125:160–70.

41. Heazell AE, Leisher S, Cregan M, et al. Sharing experiences to improve bereavement support and clinical care after stillbirth: report of the 7th annual meeting of the International Stillbirth Alliance. Acta Obstet Gynecol Scand 2013;92(3): 352–61.

42. Boyle FM, Vance JC, Najman JM, et al. The mental health impact of stillbirth, neonatal death or SIDS: prevalence and patterns of distress among mothers. Soc Sci Med 1996;43:1273–82.
43. Gold KJ, Kuznia AL, Hayward RA. How physicians cope with stillbirth or neonatal death: a national survey of obstetricians. Obstet Gynecol 2008;112:29–34.
44. Sharma PP, Salihu HM, Kirby RS. Stillbirth recurrence in a population of relatively low-risk mothers. Paediatr Perinat Epidemiol 2007;21(Suppl. 1):24–30.
45. Lamont K, Scott NW, Jones GT, et al. Risk of recurrent stillbirth: systematic review and meta-analysis. BMJ 2015;250:h3080.
46. McPherson E. Recurrence of stillbirth and second trimester pregnancy loss. Am J Med Genet A 2016;170A:1174–80.
47. Reddy UM. Prediction and prevention of recurrent stillbirth. Obstet Gynecol 2007; 110:1151–64.
48. Heuser CC, McFadden M, Hammer A, et al. Stillbirth gestational age as a predictor of recurrence risk. Am J Perinatal 2014;31:393–400.
49. Wojcieszek AM, Boyle FM, Belizan JM, et al. Care in subsequent pregnancies following stillbirth: an international survey of parents. BJOG 2018;125:193–201.
50. Regan AK, Gissler M, Magnus MC, et al. Association between interpregnancy interval and adverse birth outcomes in women with a previous stillbirth: an international cohort study. Lancet 2019;393(10180):1527–35.
51. Page JM, Silver RM. Interventions to prevent stillbirth. Semin Fetal Neonatal Med 2017;22(3):135–45.
52. Duley L, Henderson-Smart DJ, Meher S, et al. Antiplatelet agents for preventing pre-eclampsia and its complications. Cochrane Database Syst Rev 2007;2: CD004659.
53. Low-dose aspirin use during pregnancy. ACOG Committee Opinion No. 743. American College of Obstetricians and Gynecologists. Obstet Gynecol 2018; 132:e44–52.
54. Rey E, Garneau P, David M, et al. Dalteparin for the prevention of recurrence of placental-mediated complications of pregnancy in women without thrombophilia: a pilot randomized controlled trial. J Thromb Haemost 2009;7:58e64.
55. Rodger MA, Gris JC, de Vries JI, et al, Low-Molecular-Weight Heparin for Placenta-Mediated Pregnancy Complications Study Group. Low-molecular weight heparin and recurrent placenta-mediated pregnancy complications: a meta-analysis of individual patient data from randomised controlled trials. Lancet 2016;388:2629e41.
56. American College of Obstetricians and Gynecologists. Antepartum fetal surveillance. Practice Bulletin No. 145. Obstet Gynecol 2014;124:182e92.
57. Freeman RK, Anderson G, Dorchester W. A prospective multi-institutional study of antepartum fetal heart rate monitoring. I. Risk of perinatal mortality and morbidity according to antepartum fetal heart rate test results. Am J Obstet Gynecol 1982; 143:771e7.
58. Manning FA, Morrison I, Harman CR, et al. Fetal assessment based on fetal biophysical profile scoring: experience in 19,221 referred high-risk pregnancies. II. An analysis of false-negative fetal deaths. Am J Obstet Gynecol 1987;157:880e4.
59. Miller DA, Rabello YA, Paul RH. The modified biophysical profile: antepartum testing in the 1990s. Am J Obstet Gynecol 1996;174:812e7.
60. Spong CY, Mercer BM, D'Alton M, et al. Timing of indicated late-preterm and early-term birth. Obstet Gynecol 2011;118:323e33.

Post-Traumatic Stress Disorder and Severe Maternal Morbidity

Maria J. Small, MD, MPH[a,b,*],
Kaboni W. Gondwe, PhD, GH, UCM, RN[c,d], Haywood L. Brown, MD[e,f]

KEYWORDS

- Postpartum • Obstetric maternal near-miss mortality • Traumatic childbirth
- Post-traumatic stress • Racial disparities

KEY POINTS

- Approximately 9% of women have PTSD following childbirth.
- Severe maternal morbidity can trigger PTSD.
- Postpartum evaluation provides an opportunity for screening for PTSD.
- Lack of postpartum follow-up for maternal near miss impacts long-term health and adversely contributes to health disparities.

INTRODUCTION

Maternal mortality and severe maternal morbidity (SMM) have increased over the last decade in the United States.[1,2] The estimated increase in SMM is 45% from 2005 to 2016.[3,4] Maternal mortalities in the United States are fortunately rare but the challenge remains for racial disparity between non-Hispanic black women and white women. Black women are three to four times more like to die from pregnancy-related causes compared with white women and maternal mortality is higher in rural areas where access to quality care and providers is limited.[3,5] For every maternal death there are approximately 100 episodes of SMM or near misses.[6] Mortality is part of the continuum or sequelae of events that begin as severe morbidity or near misses.[7,8]

[a] Department of Obstetrics and Gynecology, Duke University, Durham, NC, USA; [b] Division of Maternal Fetal Medicine, Duke University School of Medicine, Duke University Medical Center, Box 3967, Durham, NC 27710, USA; [c] UW Milwaukee College of Nursing, Milwaukee, WI, USA; [d] Center for Advancing Population Science, Medical College of Wisconsin, Cunningham Hall 607, Milwaukee, WI 53211, USA; [e] Obstetrics and Gynecology, University of South Florida, 13101 Bruce B Downs Boulevard, Tampa, FL 33612, USA; [f] Diversity, Morsani College of Medicine, University South Florida, 13101 Bruce B Downs Boulevard, Tampa, FL 33612, USA
* Corresponding author. Division of Maternal Fetal Medicine, Duke University School of Medicine, Duke University Medical Center, Box 3967, Durham, NC 27710.
E-mail address: Maria.small@duke.edu

Obstet Gynecol Clin N Am 47 (2020) 453–461
https://doi.org/10.1016/j.ogc.2020.04.004
0889-8545/20/© 2020 Elsevier Inc. All rights reserved.

obgyn.theclinics.com

SMMs are much more common than maternal mortality.[6] Approximately 1200 maternal deaths occur annually compared with 60,000 SMMs. As such, the higher numbers of SMM allows for more robust study for a direct examination of the cascade of events; system, community, and patient level factors that may ultimately prevent or lead to the sequelae of maternal death.[6,8] Study of SMM also allows survivors to provide their accounts and perspectives on factors leading to the adverse pregnancy outcome.[9,10] SMMs are catastrophic obstetric events characterized as near misses for maternal death that might have resulted in death but the woman survives because of heroic interventions or chance.[11] SMMs are defined by disease definitions and outcomes, such as eclampsia, renal failure, severe postpartum hemorrhage, and cardiac arrest; or therapy-based, such as intensive care unit admission or massive transfusion. In many situations the categories overlap.[6,11]

Similar to maternal mortality, inequities in SMM exist with non-Hispanic black, indigenous, rural, and low-income women having higher rates of SMM compared with non-Hispanic white women in the United States.[3,5,8] From 2007 to 2016, the Centers for Disease Control and Prevention reported pregnancy-related mortality ratios for African American and American Indian/Alaska Native women at approximately 2.8 to 3.3 and 1.7 to 3.3 times higher than for non-Hispanic white women in the United States.[3] Maternal deaths are noted to be four to five times higher for African American and American Indian/Alaskan Native women greater than or equal to 30 years of age compared with white women in the same age group.[3] The racial and ethnic disparities persist despite many studies controlling for the social and demographic factors associated with adverse outcomes, prompting many authors to query whether such factors as maternal stress and structural inequities contribute to the residual risk for adverse outcomes. In work from Durham, North Carolina, pregnancy-related maternal mortality ratios were compared among African American, white non-Hispanic, and Hispanic women. Pregnancy-related maternal mortality ratios were higher for African American women and lowest for Hispanic women despite higher prevalence of social determinants associated with adverse pregnancy outcome (eg, later entry to prenatal care, non-English speaker, lack of insurance, lack of employment, lower level of formal education) for Hispanic women.[12] African American women had higher rates of chronic cardiovascular and medical comorbidities. When SMM was examined in the same population, SMM was higher for Hispanic women than African American and non-Hispanic white women.[13] Population-based data from New York City demonstrates higher rates of SMM for black and Hispanic women compared with white women.[14,15] Pooled data from seven states demonstrated rates of SMM as 2.1, 1.7, 1.3, and 1.2 times higher for black, American Indian/Alaska Native, Hispanic, and Asian/Pacific Islander women, respectively.[4]

Pregnancy and childbirth may lead to maternal depression and exacerbation, or triggering of mood disorder.[16] Perinatal depression, which includes the 12 months following childbirth, is a common pregnancy complication affecting one in seven women.[17] Women with adverse outcome during pregnancy have a higher risk for mental health conditions and depression.[7,18] In fact, high-risk factors for perinatal depression include previous history of depression, stressful life events, traumatic birth experiences, preterm birth with need for neonatal intensive care, birth defects, and obstetric near-miss morbidities. Risks for maternal death are increased in women with mental health disorders and depression. Suicide and drug overdose from opiates contribute to US maternal mortality. Women who experience pregnancy complications including SMM are at risk for decreased quality of life, decrease in sexual function, and fear of death in subsequent pregnancy.[7,18,19] In addition to potential adverse long-term health, mothers with untreated major mood disorders may affect breastfeeding and mother-infant attachment.[20] The association with these factors and maternal anxiety, depression, and post-traumatic stress disorder (PTSD) reflects the intergenerational impact of trauma.

PTSD is a serious psychological condition that results from exposure to a traumatic event, such as a death or risk for death.[21] The disorder results in symptoms of reliving the trauma, avoiding triggers associated with the trauma, and symptoms of excitability (sleep disorder, difficulty concentrating, irritability). Traumatic events may include childhood physical abuse, physical assault, or being threatening with a weapon. A large proportion of those with PTSD experience trauma before the age of 25 years.

Common symptoms of PTSD include: intrusive recollections of the traumatic stressor, avoidant/numbing behaviors, and hyperarousal symptoms.[21] For diagnosis PTSD symptoms must be present for at least a month. If symptoms persist for longer than 3 months the condition is considered chronic.

It is not difficult to understand that women with an obstetric SMM might be at higher risk for PTSD. More than one-third of mothers in the United States describe childbirth as a traumatic experience.[22] The prevalence of PTSD in women of childbearing age is approximately 10% to 13%.[23] Pregnancy and childbirth has been identified as a potential trigger for PTSD.[24] Approximately 9% of women are diagnosed with PTSD postpartum in the United States.[22,24] PTSD may follow pregnancies with normal maternal and neonatal birth outcomes. It is also known to be associated with some adverse outcomes. For instance, following a perinatal loss, stillbirth, or preterm birth, the prevalence of PTSD has been reported to be 15% to 25%.[20] Perinatal PTSD is associated with depression, preterm birth, poor mother-baby attachment, lack of breastfeeding, and later psychological symptoms.[24] PTSD in the acute and chronic forms has been associated with an increased risk for spontaneous preterm birth.[19]

PTSD in the perinatal period may result from antepartum, intrapartum, and postpartum risk factors.[25] Although not a formal Diagnostic and Statistical Manual of Mental Disorders (DSM) classification, "perinatal PTSD" is a term that may best describe the nature of the condition for the obstetric population as not solely a result of traumatic birth but potentially encompassing the entire perinatal period.[24]

Antenatal risk factors for PTSD are prior history of depression, anxiety, fear of childbirth, previous poor pregnancy outcomes, and prior history of trauma including history of abuse. Intrapartum factors associated with PTSD include maternal pain, feeling of loss of control during birth, disassociation, and poor support during labor and childbirth. Emergency cesarean birth, operative vaginal delivery, and neonatal complications also contribute to the risk for PTSD. Clearly, cesarean birth, unplanned hysterectomy perhaps because of severe hemorrhage, and loss of future childbearing are near-miss experiences that would put a woman at increased risk for PTSD. Black mothers have also shown a higher risk of PTSD than mothers from other racial backgrounds.[26] Infant condition at birth has also been shown to trigger maternal PTSD symptoms (**Table 1**).[26]

PTSD may be associated with poor maternal coping and higher stress postpartum. Depression may be present as a comorbidity, significantly increasing the risk for suicide.[25]

SMM or a near miss, by definition, represents a threat to the physical life of a woman and, in many cases, her infant. This experience could trigger PTSD. An expanding body of literature links perinatal PTSD with these potentially traumatic, life-threatening events. In addition to depression, PTSD may represent another critical condition to identify in the postpartum period. Unrecognized and untreated, perinatal PTSD may increase the risk for long-term symptoms and potential sequelae for the woman and her family.[17,27,28]

Table 1	
Risk factors for PTSD	
Antenatal	**Intrapartum and Postpartum Events**
Prior history of PTSD	Maternal pain
Prior history of depression and/or anxiety	Feeling of loss of control during birth
Prior history of trauma, including abuse	Disassociation
	Poor support during labor and birth
	Emergency cesarean delivery
	Severe maternal morbidity, "near miss"
	Poor infant outcomes

SEVERE MATERNAL MORBIDITY AND POST-TRAUMATIC STRESS DISORDER

Recent reviews and literature evaluate the association between PTSD and SMM. The literature is limited on whether the type of SMM experienced has a greater impact on the development of PTSD. Many studies in the literature do exclude pregnancy loss, because this event is known to be a high-risk factor for PTSD and maternal mood disorder.[29] However, some evidence show that women who had SMM reported higher PTSD symptoms compared with those who did not experience SMM.[30,31]

Preeclampsia is associated with an increased risk for PTSD. The prevalence of PTSD among women with preeclampsia up to 2 years postpartum ranges from 5% to 44%.[29] These data compare with approximately 3% to 7% measured between 6 weeks to a year postpartum in general populations during similar time periods.[29,32] Hoedjes and coworkers[33] examined PTSD at 6 and 12 weeks in women with preeclampsia and found significantly lower prevalence of PTSD in women with mild preeclampsia (3%) compared with women with severe preeclampsia (11%). The prevalence of PTSD symptoms (intrusion, avoidance, and hyperarousal) was higher for women with severe preeclampsia at 6 weeks and 12 weeks postpartum. Engelhard and coworkers[34] also examined prevalence of PTSD in women with preterm and term preeclampsia. The findings showed that 28% of women with preterm birth and preterm preeclampsia had PTSD compared with 17% of women with term preeclampsia and 0% of women with uncomplicated term deliveries. Stramrood and coworkers[35] compared prevalence of PTSD in mothers with preeclampsia/HELLP syndrome and preterm premature rupture of membranes at term at 6 weeks and 15 months postpartum. Findings showed a higher prevalence of PTSD in mothers with preterm premature rupture of membranes at 17% compared with 11% in preeclampsia/HELLP syndrome and 3% in uneventful term pregnancies. When excluding mothers whose infants had died the differences between group were no longer significant. This speaks to the fact that perinatal loss is a confounder for PTSD in women with other pregnancy complications, such as preeclampsia. A study from a low-income country also shows a significant relationship between psychological stress and SMM to be mediated by perinatal loss.[18]

Lewkowitz and colleagues[36] used the Florida Health Care Cost and Utilization Project database to examine singleton deliveries from 2005 to 2015 to compare composite psychiatric morbidity (suicide attempt, depression, anxiety, PTSD, psychosis, acute stress reaction, or adjustment disorder) in women with SMM with those without SMM as determined within 1 year of hospital discharge. The study demonstrated 2.9% (n = 452) of women with SMM having psychiatric morbidity compared with 1.6% of women (n= 19, 279) without SMM having psychiatric morbidity (adjusted odds ratio, 1.74; 95% confidence interval, 1.58–1.91). The highest risk interval for psychiatric morbidity was within 4 months of discharge after childbirth. Women with SMM had nearly two-fold increased risk of postpartum substance use disorder. Although, the overall sample size is robust the percent of women with PTSD and SMM (n = 11; 0.07%) compared with those without SMM and PTSD in the study was small.[36]

PERINATAL POST-TRAUMATIC STRESS DISORDER RECOGNITION AND TREATMENT

The American College of Obstetricians and Gynecologists recommends screening all women postpartum for depression and anxiety and provide individualized care with in-person visits as needed during 3 months postpartum and throughout the interpregnancy interval.[17,36,37] It is particularly important that depression screening be conducted by 3 weeks postpartum as recommended by the published postpartum guidelines for those women at high risk for depression, such as those with near-miss obstetric events.[17] However, no routine screening is done for PTSD, which limits the understanding of trauma related to childbirth complications.

For a patient to be diagnosed with PTSD the symptoms must persist for at least a month and have a negative impact on daily life. The two most commonly used screening tools for perinatal PTSD are the Traumatic Event Scale and the Perinatal PTSD questionnaire. The Traumatic Event Scale (based on DSM, fourth edition) is used in pregnancy to measure PTSD related to upcoming birth or after birth to measure PTSD in response to birth events.[38] However, Ayers and coworkers[39] argue that although the Traumatic Events Scale has good face validity research has not examined its psychometric properties against clinical interviews. The perinatal PTSD questionnaire was developed for use in high-risk moms; the modified version, a 14-item scale, does not ask about stressor criteria or cover all diagnostic criteria but does cover avoidance, intrusions, arousal, and negative cognition and mood.[29]

The City Birth Trauma Scale was revised according to DSM, fifth edition, diagnostic criteria. The City Birth Trauma Scale is a 29-item questionnaire that evaluates PTSD related to pregnancy and childbirth. The scale evaluates symptoms of re-experiencing the events, avoidance, negative mood, hyperarousal, duration of symptoms, degree of distress by frequency of symptoms ("not at all, 0–5 or more times"), and disability/distress ("yes/no/maybe"). Higher scores indicate higher symptoms.[39] Initial questions assess helplessness, fear, and hopelessness ("Did you believe you or your baby would be seriously injured during birth or did you believe you or your baby would die?"). Symptom assessment may include questions about recurrent memories, dreams, or flashbacks about events at the birth or puerperium afterward, and degree of symptoms that may have worsened since birth. Others include questions regarding feeling negative, irritable, detached/like in a dream, or self-destructive. Total possible scores are from 0 to 56. If other conditions are ruled out and the duration of symptoms is 1 month or more, findings are consistent with PTSD.[39]

The Posttraumatic Diagnostics Scale for DSM, fifth edition, is a 24-item self-report instrument that follows all the criteria of the DSM, fifth edition, and is used to measure PTSD symptoms during the most recent month.[40] The instrument has two items that initially screen a person's history of trauma followed by 20 items that examine presence and severity of PTSD symptoms and four items that explore distress and interference as a result of PTSD symptoms and the onset and duration of those symptoms. The Posttraumatic Diagnostics Scale for DSM, fifth edition, has been tested for use in postpartum mothers and showed high internal consistency and high concurrent validity for measuring postpartum psychopathology.[41]

Therapies for PTSD typically begin with cognitive behavioral intervention with a trauma focus, trauma-focused cognitive behavioral therapy, and eye movement desensitization.[42,43] Serotonin reuptake inhibitors, such as sertraline and venlafaxine, are also effective and may be used alone or in combination with psychotherapy.[44] Medication may be effective as a first-line approach if patients prefer or if cognitive behavioral therapy is not available. Patients should remain on serotonin reuptake inhibitors for 6 months to a year to prevent relapse. Counseling and debriefing may be helpful to patients with stress responses to SMMs.[20] Social support in the perinatal period could also promote maternal confidence and consequently lower the risk for PTSD.[22]

SUMMARY

SMM has been associated with PTSD. Although small, an increasing body of literature examines the potential direct association between PTSD and SMM.[29] The recognition of PTSD and other mood disorders following SMM may lessen the long-term impact of these conditions on long-term health and the potential impact on current children and future pregnancies. Ideally, counseling should be grounded in a trauma-based approach.

It is critical that women with SMM have postpartum guidance so that they have the opportunity to be evaluated for PTSD because they are at higher risk for posttraumatic stress.[37] The prevention of PTSD or reduction of severity of symptoms also requires early detection of risk factors and provision of support throughout pregnancy and childbirth and the postpartum period.[22] Traumatic delivery, cesarean hysterectomy for severe hemorrhage, and subsequent loss of future reproduction is potentially a major risk factor. The clinician must be aware of the risk factors for PTSD as related to near misses and provide the appropriate avenues for counseling and follow-up within the 12 months following childbirth. Women with an obstetric near miss represent those with a unique circumstance that places them at greater risk for adverse outcome in a subsequent pregnancy. These findings further emphasize the potential beneficial impact of counseling during the interpregnancy interval to mitigate against recurrence. Furthermore, it emphasizes the need for a follow-up preconception visit to discuss risk for recurrence and to address anxieties for future childbirth and strategies for prevention of obstetric complications. This is especially relevant for women in their 40s who may or may not have experienced NMM after in vitro fertilization and contemplating another pregnancy through in vitro fertilization or embryo transfer. By virtue of age alone they are at higher risk for recurrence of obstetric complications, morbidity, and mortality.[45] Promoting perinatal support should also be key in management of women with obstetric complications because this would promote maternal mental health and reduce the severity of the PTSD experience.

DISCLOSURE

Authors have nothing to disclose.

REFERENCES

1. Petersen EE, Davis NL, Goodman D, et al. Vital Signs: Pregnancy-Related Deaths, United States, 2011–2015, and Strategies for Prevention, 13 States, 2013–2017. MMWR Morbidity and Mortality Weekly Report 2019;68(18).

2. Creanga AA, Callaghan WM. Recent increases in the U.S. maternal mortality rate: disentangling trends from measurement issues. Obstet Gynecol 2017;129(1): 206–7.

3. Petersen EE, Davis NL, Goodman D, et al. Racial/ethnic disparities in pregnancy-related deaths—United States, 2007-2016. MMWR Morb Mortal Wkly Rep 2019; 68(35):762–5.

4. Creanga AA, Bateman BT, Kuklina EV, et al. Racial and ethnic disparities in severe maternal morbidity: a multistate analysis, 2008-2010. Am J Obstet Gynecol 2014;210(5):435.e1-8.

5. Kozhimannil KB, Interrante JD, Henning-Smith C, et al. Rural-urban differences in severe maternal morbidity and mortality in the US, 2007-15. Health Aff (Millwood) 2019;38(12):2077–85.

6. Callaghan WM, Creanga AA, Kuklina EV. Severe maternal morbidity among delivery and postpartum hospitalizations in the United States. Obstet Gynecol 2012; 120(5):1029–36.

7. Angelini CR, Pacagnella RC, Parpinelli MA, et al. Post-traumatic stress disorder and severe maternal morbidity: is there an association? Clinics (Sao Paulo) 2018;73:e309.

8. Howell EA. Reducing disparities in severe maternal morbidity and mortality. Clin Obstet Gynecol 2018;61(2):387–99.

9. Tuncalp O, Hindin MJ, Souza JP, et al. The prevalence of maternal near miss: a systematic review. BJOG 2012;119(6):653–61.

10. Souza JP, Cecatti JG, Haddad SM, et al. The WHO maternal near-miss approach and the maternal severity index model (MSI): tools for assessing the management of severe maternal morbidity. PLoS One 2012;7(8):e44129.

11. Say L, Pattinson RC, Gulmezoglu AM. WHO systematic review of maternal morbidity and mortality: the prevalence of severe acute maternal morbidity (near miss). Reprod Health 2004;1(1):3.

12. Brown HL, Chireau MV, Jallah Y, et al. The "Hispanic paradox": an investigation of racial disparity in pregnancy outcomes at a tertiary care medical center. Am J Obstet Gynecol 2007;197(2):197.e1-7 [discussion: 197.e7–9].

13. Brown HL, Small M, Taylor YJ, et al. Near miss maternal mortality in a multiethnic population. Ann Epidemiol 2011;21(2):73–7.

14. Howell EA, Egorova NN, Janevic T, et al. Severe maternal morbidity among Hispanic women in New York City: investigation of health disparities. Obstet Gynecol 2017;129(2):285–94.

15. Howell EA, Egorova N, Balbierz A, et al. Black-white differences in severe maternal morbidity and site of care. Am J Obstet Gynecol 2016;214(1):122 e121–127.

16. Lancaster CA, Gold KJ, Flynn HA, et al. Risk factors for depressive symptoms during pregnancy: a systematic review. Am J Obstet Gynecol 2010;202(1):5–14.

17. ACOG Committee opinion no. 757 summary: screening for perinatal depression. Obstet Gynecol 2018;132(5):1314–6.

18. Adewuya AO, Ologun YA, Ibigbami OS. Post-traumatic stress disorder after childbirth in Nigerian women: prevalence and risk factors. BJOG 2006;113(3):284–8.

19. Shaw JG, Asch SM, Kimerling R, et al. Posttraumatic stress disorder and risk of spontaneous preterm birth. Obstet Gynecol 2014;124(6):1111–9.

20. Cunen NMJ, Murray K. A systematic review of midwife-led interventions to address post partum post-traumatic stress. Midwifery 2014;30:170–84.

21. American Psychiatric Association, American Psychiatric Association, DSM-5 Task Force. Diagnostic and statistical manual of mental disorders: DSM-5. 5th edition. Washington, DC: American Psychiatric Association; 2013.

22. Vesel J, Nickasch B. An evidence review and model for prevention and treatment of postpartum posttraumatic stress disorder. Nurs Womens Health 2015;19(6): 504–25.

23. Cook N, Ayers S, Horsch A. Maternal posttraumatic stress disorder during the perinatal period and child outcomes: a systematic review. J Affect Disord 2018; 225:18–31.

24. Vignato J, Georges JM, Bush RA, et al. Post-traumatic stress disorder in the perinatal period: a concept analysis. J Clin Nurs 2017;26(23–24):3859–68.

25. Polachek IS, Fung K, Vigod SN. First lifetime psychiatric admission in the postpartum period: a population-based comparison to women with prior psychiatric admission. Gen Hosp Psychiatry 2016;40:25–32.

26. Furuta M, Sandall J, Cooper D, et al. Predictors of birth-related post-traumatic stress symptoms: secondary analysis of a cohort study. Arch Womens Ment Health 2016;19(6):987–99.

27. Koblinsky M, Chowdhury ME, Moran A, et al. Maternal morbidity and disability and their consequences: neglected agenda in maternal health. J Health Popul Nutr 2012;30(2):124–30.

28. Filippi V, Ganaba R, Baggaley RF, et al. Health of women after severe obstetric complications in Burkina Faso: a longitudinal study. Lancet 2007;370(9595): 1329–37.

29. Furuta M, Sandall J, Bick D. A systematic review of the relationship between severe maternal morbidity and post-traumatic stress disorder. BMC Pregnancy Childbirth 2012;12:125.

30. Furuta M, Sandall J, Cooper D, et al. The relationship between severe maternal morbidity and psychological health symptoms at 6-8 weeks postpartum: a prospective cohort study in one English maternity unit. BMC Pregnancy Childbirth 2014;14:133.

31. Silveira MS, Gurgel RQ, Barreto IDC, et al. Severe maternal morbidity: posttraumatic suffering and social support. Rev Bras Enferm 2018;71(suppl 5): 2139–45.

32. Ayers S, Joseph S, McKenzie-McHarg K, et al. Post-traumatic stress disorder following childbirth: current issues and recommendations for future research. J Psychosom Obstet Gynaecol 2008;29(4):240–50.

33. Hoedjes M, Berks D, Vogel I, et al. Symptoms of post-traumatic stress after preeclampsia. J Psychosom Obstet Gynaecol 2011;32(3):126–34.

34. Engelhard IM, van Rij M, Boullart I, et al. Posttraumatic stress disorder after preeclampsia: an exploratory study. Gen Hosp Psychiatry 2002;24(4):260–4.

35. Stramrood CA, Huis In 't Veld EM, Van Pampus MG, et al. Measuring posttraumatic stress following childbirth: a critical evaluation of instruments. J Psychosom Obstet Gynaecol 2010;31(1):40–9.

36. Lewkowitz AK, Rosenbloom JI, Keller M, et al. Association between severe maternal morbidity and psychiatric illness within 1 year of hospital discharge after delivery. Obstet Gynecol 2019;134(4):695–707.

37. ACOG Committee Opinion No. 736: optimizing postpartum care. Obstet Gynecol 2018;131(5):e140–50.

38. Soderquist J, Wijma B, Thorbert G, et al. Risk factors in pregnancy for posttraumatic stress and depression after childbirth. BJOG 2009;116(5):672–80.

39. Ayers S, Wright DB, Thornton A. Development of a measure of postpartum PTSD: the city birth trauma scale. Front Psychiatry 2018;9:409.
40. Foa EB, McLean CP, Zang Y, et al. Psychometric properties of the posttraumatic stress disorder symptom scale interview for DSM-5 (PSSI-5). Psychol Assess 2016;28(10):1159–65.
41. Dikmen-Yildiz P, Ayers S, Phillips L. Screening for birth-related PTSD: psychometric properties of the Turkish version of the Posttraumatic Diagnostic Scale in postpartum women in Turkey. Eur J Psychotraumatol 2017;8(1):1306414.
42. Ursano RJ, Bell C, Eth S, et al. Practice guideline for the treatment of patients with acute stress disorder and posttraumatic stress disorder. Am J Psychiatry 2004; 161(11 Suppl):3–31.
43. Bisson JI. Post-traumatic stress disorder. Occup Med (Lond) 2007;57(6): 399–403.
44. Davidson J, Baldwin D, Stein DJ, et al. Treatment of posttraumatic stress disorder with venlafaxine extended release: a 6-month randomized controlled trial. Arch Gen Psychiatry 2006;63(10):1158–65.
45. Grotegut CA, Chisholm CA, Johnson LN, et al. Medical and obstetric complications among pregnant women aged 45 and older. PLoS One 2014;9(4):e96237.

Postpartum Contraception Options

Serina Floyd, MD, MSPH*

KEYWORDS

- Postpartum • Contraception • Counseling • Reproductive justice • Hormonal
- Nonhormonal • Breastfeeding • Sterilization

KEY POINTS

- Adequate pregnancy spacing is important to optimization of maternal and infant health.
- Conversations about contraception should begin during prenatal care visits and continue through intrapartum care and into the postpartum period.
- Contraceptive counseling should incorporate a patient-centered framework with shared medical decision making.
- A reproductive justice framework for contraceptive counseling encourages counselors to explore a person's reproductive goals, contraceptive priorities and preferences, and ability to successfully use a contraceptive method.
- Many methods of contraception are safe and effective to use in the postpartum period in order to help patients achieve their reproductive goals.

INTRODUCTION

The antenatal and postpartum periods provide unique windows during which maternal health care needs can be identified and addressed. Patients often have regular contact with a provider during prenatal visits and while hospitalized after delivery, which allows opportunities for discussion on various matters, including contraception. Many women are motivated to discuss and/or initiate contraception during this time because they often desire to prevent a rapid repeat pregnancy. In addition, for those who were previously uninsured, pregnancy and the postpartum period allow access to health care and/or insurance coverage they may not otherwise have.

Conversations about contraception should optimally begin during prenatal care visits, but can be continued through intrapartum care and into the postpartum period. As many as 40% of women do not return for a 6-week postpartum visit, so discussing contraceptive options and initiation of the desired contraceptive method before delivery are key. Reasons women do not return for the 6-week postpartum visit are varied

Planned Parenthood of Metropolitan Washington, DC, Washington, DC, USA
* PO Box 11020, Alexandria, VA 22312.
E-mail address: serina.floyd@gmail.com

Obstet Gynecol Clin N Am 47 (2020) 463–475
https://doi.org/10.1016/j.ogc.2020.04.007
0889-8545/20/© 2020 Elsevier Inc. All rights reserved.

obgyn.theclinics.com

and include lack of insurance coverage, employment restrictions, childcare obligations, lack of transportation, and communication or language barriers.[1] Evidence that non–breastfeeding women can ovulate as early as 25 days' postpartum with 40% ovulating by 6 weeks' postpartum, and that 57% become sexually active by 6 weeks' postpartum, highlights the need for contraception conversations to occur as early as possible.[2,3]

Adequate pregnancy spacing is important to optimization of maternal and infant health. Initiation of a contraceptive method is essential to the lengthening of the interpregnancy interval with the assumption of resumption of sexual activity following delivery. The minimum recommended interpregnancy interval is 18 months, and evidence supports that repeat pregnancy sooner than this can be associated with adverse outcomes. Birth intervals of less than 6 months carry higher risks of low-birth-weight infants, small-for-gestational-age infants, and preterm delivery.[4–6] Despite these findings, approximately one-third of women conceive within 18 months of a prior birth.[7,8]

COUNSELING

Contraceptive counseling should inform women about all options available to them with the objective of working toward selection of the method the individual feels will best meet their individual needs. Discussions should incorporate a patient-centered framework with shared medical decision making. Shared medical decision making is a process in which the provider shares comprehensive contraceptive information to the patient and the patient shares all relevant personal information that may make 1 method more or less desirable than another.[9,10] The components of shared decision making are included in **Box 1**. This process allows an even exchange of information that emphasizes a woman's values and preferences and as a result can ensure a positive patient-provider interaction and lead to increased patient engagement, satisfaction, and contraceptive adherence.[10–12]

Many factors contribute to patient decisions about contraception and to the ultimate initiation of a particular method (**Box 2**), emphasizing why shared decision making is important. Providers are able to review with patients the specifics of contraceptive methods, such as the risks, benefits, alternatives, side effects, efficacy, dosing, initiation, follow-up, and discontinuation. Patients may then specify what factors are most important to them, such as ease of use, length of protection, and lack of a requirement

---

Box 1
Components of shared decision making

1. Focus on interpersonal relationships, work to establish trust and openness to develop rapport

2. Elicit patient preferences for methods using open-ended questions

3. Be attuned to diverse patient preferences and understand that patients will have varied preferences around issues

4. Provide relevant information in accordance with patient preferences, prioritizing what is most important to the patient

5. Be aware of and responsive to patient preferences during counseling and adjust accordingly

Adapted from Dehlendorf C, Fox E, Sobel L, et al. Patient-centered contraceptive counseling: evidence to inform practice. Curr Obstet Gynecol Rep 2016;5:55-63; with permission.

Box 2
Factors that affect patient contraceptive use

- Medical conditions
- Patient preference
- Future pregnancy goals
- Reliability of a method
- Efficacy of a method
- Side effects
- Convenience
- Ease of use
- Ability to control method
- Safety, particular during breastfeeding
- Access to medical care
- Method cost
- Insurance coverage

Data from Cwiak C, Gellasch T, Zieman M. Peripartum contraceptive attitudes and practices. Contraception 2004;70(5):383-6.

---

for a monthly pharmacy trip. Receiving the information in both verbal and written formats, as well through the Internet, is also important to women.[10]

The prenatal period is the optimal time during which to initiate contraceptive counseling because women in the immediate postpartum period are usually focused on care of the newborn and recovery from childbirth. The prenatal period is also optimal because methods reviewed prenatally can be initiated at the time of delivery or during the hospital stay. Patients prefer to have counseling during the prenatal period.[13] However, a woman's circumstances and opinions may change over time so the discussion should be revisited intrapartum and postpartum.[14] In 1 study, 46% of postpartum women chose a different method postpartum than what they used before pregnancy.[15]

Incorporation of a Reproductive Justice Framework

The history of contraception in the United States includes many abuses perpetrated against multiple communities, particularly women of color and economically marginalized women. Abuses perpetrated under the guise of public health have included forced and coerced sterilization of institutionalized individuals, mentally and physically disabled persons, women with low incomes, women of color, indigenous women, and immigrant women during the eugenics movement of the early twentieth century. Reproductive oppression and injustices continued through the 1970s with use of sterilization, as well as other forms of contraception, as a means of punishment, as a means of extortion to ensure receipt of public assistance, under threat of deportation, and to "address" poverty and childbearing outside of marriage.[16,17] Contraceptive experimentation without informed consent on economically disadvantaged Puerto Rican women is another example of egregious abuses perpetrated against women of color. Provider awareness of this history and its potential impact on decision making for individuals is essential to ensuring respect, value, and elevation of patient desires and goals during contraceptive counseling.

The reproductive justice movement was born from recognition of historical injustices and abuses in all communities, especially communities where people of color live, and serves as the foundation for efforts to address reproductive oppression. It is rooted in human rights and was first developed by women of color in the early 1990s. The reproductive justice framework combines *reproductive rights* and *social justice* and highlights the intersections of race, class, and gender. Reproductive justice uplifts and centers the unique lived experiences and concerns of marginalized peoples in the broader reproductive choice and rights movement and highlights women's ability to exercise self-determination and bodily autonomy. The framework has the following 3 primary principles: (1) the right to not have a child; (2) the right to have a child; and (3) the right to parent children in safe and healthy environments.[18,19]

A reproductive justice framework for contraceptive counseling encourages counselors to explore a person's reproductive goals, contraceptive priorities and preferences, and ability to successfully use a contraceptive method. The ability to successfully initiate and continue a contraceptive method may include such factors as health literacy, socioeconomic status, race, ethnicity, religious beliefs, insurance status, age, sexual minority status, mental health, substance use, and other factors. Providers must also acknowledge the systemic and structural barriers that may impede an individual's ability to use their preferred method.[18,19]

Incorporating reproductive justice into contraceptive care also means providers must examine issues of personal bias regarding an individual's contraceptive decisions and reproductive goals that may be affecting provider-patient interactions. Biases may be implicit and can present as thoughts about whether or when individuals should or should not have children. Practices such as overemphasizing long-acting reversible contraception over short-acting methods for certain women from marginalized populations, including those who qualify for Medicaid or for programs for free devices, targets economically disadvantaged women for provider-controlled contraception. All options should be reviewed equally to all patients, and the method the *patient* selects should be respected. Increasing access to care should be the focus rather than increasing uptake of a particular method. Resist potential coercion by avoiding judgment or pressure to initiate a particular contraceptive method. Respect reproductive autonomy and when possible advocate for equitable access and change.

POSTPARTUM CONTRACEPTIVE INITIATION, SAFETY, AND METHODS
Postpartum Initiation/Safety/Breastfeeding Considerations

The 2016 US Medical Eligibility Criteria for Contraceptive Use published by the Centers for Disease Control and Prevention provides guidelines for the safe use of contraceptive methods by individuals with certain characteristics or known preexisting medical conditions. Each condition or characteristic receives a category rating for every contraceptive method that ranges from 1 (no restrictions for use) to 4 (unacceptable health risk if the contraceptive method is used) (**Box 3**).

Specific guidelines exist for the initiation of contraception during the postpartum period. Breastfeeding status is a key consideration, but even in the absence of breastfeeding, increased risk of postpartum venous thromboembolism (VTE) guides recommendations regarding initiation of estrogen-containing methods. Regardless of breastfeeding status, high risk of VTE during the first 21 days after delivery results

---

Box 3
Categories of medical eligibility criteria for contraceptive use classification

1. A condition for which there is no restriction for the use of the contraceptive method
2. A condition for which the advantages of using the method generally outweigh the theoretic or proven risks
3. A condition for which the theoretic or proven risks usually outweigh the advantages of using the method
4. A condition that represents an unacceptable health risk if the contraceptive method is used

Modified from Centers for Disease Control and Prevention (CDC). Summary chart of U.S. medical eligibility criteria for contraceptive use. 2010. Available at: http://www.cdc.gov/reproductivehealth/unintendedpregnancy/pdf/legal_summary-chart_english_final_tag508.pdf. Accessed Dec 20 2019.

---

in the recommendation that combined hormonal methods (methods that contain both estrogen and progestin) not be used during this time because the health risks are unacceptable (category 4). During the period of 21 to 42 days' postpartum, in the absence of other risks for VTE (age $\geq$35, previous VTE, thrombophilia, immobility, transfusion at delivery, peripartum cardiomyopathy, body mass index [BMI] $\geq$30 kg/m^2, postpartum hemorrhage, post–cesarean delivery, preeclampsia, or smoking), combined hormonal methods are acceptable (category 2). In the presence of those risks, combined methods are category 3. Beyond 42 days' postpartum, non–breastfeeding individuals with no other medical contraindications have no restrictions on combined methods (category 1).[20]

The guidelines for breastfeeding women vary slightly from those of non–breastfeeding women. Recommendations are based on evidence of potential negative effects of the estrogen component of hormonal contraception on breastfeeding duration and success, in addition to VTE risk. For women less than 21 days' postpartum, the category rating remains 4 for combined methods, but between 21 days' and 30 days' postpartum, both with and without the above-mentioned VTE risk factors, combined hormonal methods are category 3. For patients who are past 30 days' postpartum but with VTE risk factors, use of combined methods are rated category 3. Without VTE risks, the rating improves to 2. Once past 42 days' postpartum, combined methods are acceptable to use with no restrictions in breastfeeding women (category 2).

Progestin-only hormonal options (pills, contraceptive injection, contraceptive implant, and the levonorgestrel [LNG] intrauterine device [IUD]) and most nonhormonal methods (copper IUD [Cu-IUD], male and female condoms, lactational amenorrhea [LAM], and withdrawal) may be initiated immediately postpartum in both breastfeeding and non–breastfeeding women. All types are designated category 1 or 2. The only exception is in the case of puerperal sepsis, when neither type of IUD should be initiated because they are rated category 4. The diaphragm and cervical cap should not be used until 6 weeks' postpartum at which time they become category 1.

Hormonal Contraceptive Methods

Hormonal contraception includes combined hormonal methods (methods that include estrogen and progestins) and progestin-only methods. The combined methods include oral contraceptive pills (OCPs), the transdermal contraceptive patch, and the contraceptive vaginal ring. The progestin-only methods include an oral contraceptive pill, the intramuscular or subcutaneous injection, the subdermal implant, and LNG IUDs.

Combined hormonal contraception

Combined hormonal contraceptive methods (**Table 1**) primarily contain ethinyl estradiol (EE) in varying doses and administration routes along with one of several progestins. Each method has distinct features that may make it more or less favorable to patients so a review of each option is important. All methods are highly effective when used consistently and correctly.[21] Each offers similar benefits and risks to the others. These methods should not be initiated until after a minimum of 21 days' postpartum because of the additive effect of the inherent risk of VTE with estrogen-containing contraceptives combined with the elevated VTE risk of the postpartum state. The risk for VTE is highest during the first 3 weeks' postpartum.

Formulations of OCPs contain between 10 and 35 μg of EE with varying dosages of progestins and can be monophasic (containing the same amount of hormones in each active tablet) or multiphasic (containing varying amounts of progestin or estrogen in the active pills). Regimens can be cyclic, extended, or continuous, depending on a patient's preference for frequency of withdrawal bleeding.

The transdermal contraceptive patch contains EE and norelgestromin. A higher overall concentration of EE in patch users may result in an increased risk of thromboembolism, so careful consideration of a patient's health history, including the postpartum state, must be given. Because the patch is placed topically, individuals with dermatologic disorders or skin hypersensitivity to components of the patch should avoid this method.

Table 1
Combined hormonal contraceptive methods

Method	Typical Use Effectiveness, %	Mechanism of Action	Special Considerations
OCPs	91	• Ovulation suppression • Cervical mucus thickening • Alteration of the endometrium	• Must be taken same time every day • Efficacy can be affected by certain medications
Transdermal patch	91	Same as OCPs	• Placed on skin once weekly for 3 wk then removed for 1 wk (avoid breasts) • May not be as effective in obese patients • May be associated with higher thromboembolic risk • May detach from skin
Vaginal ring	91	Same as OCPs	• Placed in vagina for 3 wk then removed for 1 wk • If bothersome during sex can remove for up to 3 h • Requires refrigeration for storage (except the segesterone acetate–containing ring)

The contraceptive vaginal ring contains EE and etonogestrel (commercial name NuvaRing, EluRyng) or segesterone acetate (commercial name Annovera). The EE/segesterone acetate ring is a 1-year reusable ring that is worn for 3 weeks and removed for 1 week and then is reused in the same manner for a total of 13 cycles. The device is latex free and can be used with water-based vaginal medications should treatment of a gynecologic condition be needed, but should not be used with oil-based medications because these have been associated with increased hormone levels. In such instances, oral medical therapies are advised instead.[22,23]

Noncontraceptive benefits In addition to contraceptive benefits, combined hormonal methods also have multiple noncontraceptive benefits. They are often prescribed for treatment of heavy menstrual bleeding or dysmenorrhea because they are effective in reducing menstrual blood loss and uterine cramping. They are prescribed for treatment of pain related to endometriosis, to control ovarian cyst formation, and for treatment of acne and premenstrual symptoms. These conditions may not present in the immediate postpartum timeframe but may begin, or return, in later postpartum months. With use, patients also receive the benefits of decreased risk of endometrial and ovarian cancer, and a reduction in risk of colorectal cancer.[24]

Progestin-only contraception
Progestin-only contraception includes methods with various delivery systems, such as progestin-only OCPs, the contraceptive injection (with an intramuscular route and a patient-administered subcutaneous route), the subdermal implant, and the IUDs (**Table 2**). All of these methods are particularly favorable for individuals with contraindications to estrogen, and all are safe for immediate postpartum use, in both breastfeeding and non–breastfeeding women. The progestin type is different for each method (norethindrone for the pills, medroxyprogesterone acetate in the injection, etonogestrel in the implant, and LNG in the IUD), but all are safe postpartum. There are 4 different LNG IUDs that vary in size, hormonal content, and duration of use. The 52-mg LNG IUDs are manufactured by different pharmaceutical companies and include Mirena and Liletta. Liletta has a Food and Drug Administration (FDA)-approved duration of 6 years as of October 2019, whereas Mirena is FDA approved for 5 years. There is evidence that both methods provide effective contraception for 7 years.[25,26] The other 2 devices include a 19.5-mg LNG device, Kyleena, and a 13.5-mg device, Skyla. These devices are smaller in size than the 52-mg devices and are approved for 5 years and 3 years, respectively. These devices should not be extended beyond the FDA-approved timeframe.

Nonhormonal Contraception

The nonhormonal contraceptive method category includes a variety of options with differing mechanisms of action, requirements for correct use, and efficacy. This group consists of the Cu-IUD, barrier methods (male and female condoms, cervical cap, diaphragm, and contraceptive sponge), LAM, fertility awareness-based methods (FABMs), and withdrawal. These options are particularly favorable for individuals with medical conditions that increase the risk of hormonal methods.

The Cu-IUD is a highly effective method with typical use effectiveness of greater than 99%.[21] Its mechanism of action is through inhibition of sperm migration and viability. The Cu-IUD currently available in the United States has FDA approval for 10 years of use, but evidence supports use for 12 years.[27] In addition to being one of the most effective forms of contraception, it is also the most effective method of emergency contraception (EC).

Table 2
Progestin-only contraceptive methods

Method	Typical Use Effectiveness, %	Mechanism of Action	Special Considerations
OCPs	91	• Thickening of cervical mucus • Ovulation suppression in only 57% of cycles	• Must be taken within 3 h of the same time each day
Contraceptive injection	94	• Ovulation suppression • Cervical mucus thickening • Alteration of the endometrium	• Can be administered intramuscularly (in clinic) or subcutaneously (by patient) every 3 mo • Most women become amenorrheic over time • Improves seizure control • Decreases sickle cell crisis • Can cause bone loss • Can cause weight gain • Unpredictable return to fertility
Subdermal implant	>99	• Ovulation suppression • Cervical mucus thickening • Alteration of the endometrium	• Placed subdermally in nondominant arm • Changes in bleeding pattern are common • FDA approval for 3 y but evidence supports 5 y[26] • Must be placed by trained clinician who attended the manufacturer training
IUD	>99	• Prevents fertilization by altering amount and viscosity of cervical mucus	• Most women ovulate normally • Must be placed by a trained clinician • 4 different devices

Male and female condoms, the diaphragm, cervical cap, and contraceptive sponge are all barrier methods that require proper placement before every act of intercourse. Condoms, with an efficacy rate of 82%,[21] may be used as soon as coitus resumes postpartum and have the added advantage of protection against sexually transmitted infections. Female condoms are made of polyurethane or nitrile and are positioned so the closed ring is inserted to cover the cervix and the open end sits outside the vagina, covering the vulva. Efficacy of the diaphragm is 88%; efficacy of the cervical cap is 71% to 86%, and efficacy of the birth control sponge is 76% to 88%.[21] These methods work by covering the cervix to serve as a barrier to sperm. The diaphragm and cervical cap may need to be fitted by a health care provider; both require a pre-scription, and both are used with spermicide to maximize effectiveness. All three of these barrier options must be placed before initiating penile-vaginal sexual activity and must be left in place between 6 to 24 hours after intercourse. The diaphragm, cervical cap, and contraceptive sponge should not be used until 6 weeks' postpartum when pregnancy-related cervical changes resolve and bleeding has diminished, mandating an alternative contraceptive method if sexual activity resumes before then. Locating carriers of these options may present a challenge because they are not always available at local pharmacies.

LAM can be a highly effective contraceptive method when used correctly, but it is a temporary method. The following 3 conditions must be met for LAM:

- The woman must be less than 6 months postpartum
- The infant must be exclusively or nearly exclusive breastfeeding, frequently with day and night feedings
- The woman must be amenorrheic

If all 3 criteria are met, efficacy can be as high as 98%.

FABMs use signs and symptoms to predict fertile days in a menstrual cycle and hence when unprotected coitus should be avoided. These methods are used primarily by couples who prefer a more "natural" pregnancy prevention method. There are multiple ways to track fertility through FABMs, including calendar tracking, basal body temperature charting, luteinizing hormone (LH) surge kits, and cervical mucus testing. There are also many computer and cell phone applications that can track this information, making the process more convenient than in the past. This method may be challenging to use in the immediate postpartum period because there is required lead time to assess cycle regularity. Breastfeeding and the physiologic hormonal return to baseline may cause cycles to be irregular or unpredictable. FABMs do require partner cooperation, as well as regular menstrual cycles with daily tracking. Efficacy is 76%.[21]

Finally, withdrawal is a method of contraception that is free, nonhormonal, and readily available, but one which also requires partner cooperation and consistent use. Efficacy is 78%.[21] Care must be taken with this method as preejaculate may contain sperm in very low numbers that could still result in pregnancy.

Immediate Postpartum Intrauterine Device Placement

Immediate postpartum placement of an IUD is the placement of an LNG or Cu-IUD within the first 48 hours of delivery. Immediate *postplacental* placement refers to placement within 10 minutes of placental delivery, which is a safe and effective time to initiate intrauterine contraception. Many women are motivated for this option immediately following delivery because pregnancy is excluded, both the provider and the patient are present, the need for additional visits presenting potential access issues is eliminated, and for those whose insurance coverage is time limited, the potential loss of insurance is avoided. Satisfaction rates are high as are continuation rates. In 1 study, 74% of women who had an IUD placed immediately postpartum still had the IUD in place 1 year later.[28]

Most patients are appropriate candidates for immediate postpartum insertion. There are no additional contraindications over interval placement with the exception of uterine infection related to delivery and ongoing hemorrhage.[20] A primary concern presents around expulsion rates, which are noted to be higher than with interval insertion. There is wide variability in reported expulsion rates ranging from 0% to 27% depending on the study, device type, and route of delivery. This rate is compared with 0% to 11% with interval placement.[29] Despite this risk, for patients with barriers to interval placement, the advantages of immediate placement may outweigh the risks. Using shared decision making, patients should be counseled about the increased risk, and if she desires to proceed, insertion should occur with specific instruction to contact her provider or return for follow-up if expulsion is suspected or confirmed. Following the paradigm for a postpartum visit with a provider within the first 3 weeks after childbirth, women with immediate postpartum contraception are obvious candidates to return for an evaluation to check for proper placement, for expulsion of an IUD, or for signs and symptoms that might suggest concerns. If the IUD has been expelled, the patient may have another device placed at that visit if she desires to continue with this method.

Emergency Contraception

EC is a drug or device used following unprotected or inadequately protected intercourse to reduce risk of pregnancy. Types include LNG-containing pills (available over the counter), ulipristal acetate (requires prescription), the Yuzpe method (a combination of 100 μg EE and 0.5 mg LNG achieved by use of any brand of combined oral contraceptives), and the Cu-IUD. LNG-containing pills, ulipristal acetate, and the Yuzpe method all work by delaying ovulation if taken at the appropriate time in the menstrual cycle. They will not prevent ovulation if taken after the LH surge, nor will they prevent implantation, and it is important to dispel any myths that they are abortifacients because they have no postfertilization effects. They should be taken as soon as possible after an act of unprotected or inadequately protected intercourse but may be taken up to 120 hours later. The Cu-IUD works primarily by impairing motility, viability, and acrosomal reaction of sperm. It is the most effective method of EC, regardless of BMI, and is also a good option for the patient who desires ongoing contraception. It should also be placed as soon as possible but may be placed up to 5 days after an act of inadequately protected intercourse.[30]

Unprotected intercourse before 21 days' postpartum does not likely need EC.[31] Beyond day 21, LNG methods of EC may be used in the postpartum period regardless of breastfeeding status, but the Cu-IUD should be inserted after 4 weeks' postpartum. There are little data on the safety of ulipristal acetate with breastfeeding.[32]

Postpartum Sterilization

Postpartum tubal sterilization is one of the safest and most effective methods of contraception with a typical use failure rate of less than 1%.[21] It is also one of the most popular over many decades, relied on by 25% of women aged 15 to 44 for prevention of pregnancy.[33] The immediate postpartum period is a convenient time to perform the procedure for the patient and can be performed with relative technical ease by the physician at the time of cesarean delivery. After vaginal delivery, postpartum sterilization can be performed through a small incision under the same regional anesthesia used for labor and delivery. The technique typically involves partial tubal excision but can also involve application of Filshie clips.

Despite the convenience in timing, only 39% to 57% of women who request postpartum sterilization during prenatal contraception counseling actually undergo the procedure,[34–37] and successful completion is lower after vaginal delivery than cesarean birth.[38] Unfulfilled sterilization procedures during hospitalization following delivery have significant consequences because nearly one-half of women who do not undergo the procedure become pregnant again within 1 year.[39] Multiple barriers exist including lack of available operating room space, surgical or anesthesia staff, lack of timely completion or presence of federal consent forms, provider-related factors (concern for young age and possible regret, low parity, competing clinical demands, insurance status, or personal religious beliefs), negative patient-provider interactions, maternal medical conditions, or receiving care in a religiously affiliated hospital.[40] In some cases, procedures go unfulfilled because of a patient's decision to delay or cancel the procedure.[36,41] Regardless of the reason, providers and hospital systems should work to identify individual and environmental obstacles to postpartum sterilization in order to eliminate barriers to care for patients.

SUMMARY

Pregnancy and the postpartum period are ideal times for health care providers to identify and address the contraceptive needs and desires of their patients. In addition to the opportunity to promote healthy pregnancy spacing, individuals can also be cared for at a time when it is convenient, there is access to health care, and motivation to prevent repeat pregnancy is high. Patient-centered care using a shared decision-making framework can not only promote positive patient-provider interactions but also increase positive outcomes.

DISCLOSURE

S. Floyd trains providers in Nexplanon insertion and removal.

REFERENCES

1. Bryant A, Haas J, McElrath T, et al. Predictors of compliance with the postpartum visit among women living in healthy start project areas. Matern Child Health J 2006;10:511–6.
2. Gray R, Campbell O, Zacur H, et al. Postpartum return of ovarian activity in non-breastfeeding women monitored by urinary assays. J Clin Endocrinol Metab 1987;64:645–50.
3. Connolly A, Thorp J, Pahel L. Effects of pregnancy and childbirth on postpartum sexual function: a longitudinal prospective study. Int Urogynecol J Pelvic Floor Dysfunct 2005;16:263–7.
4. Interpregnancy care. Obstetric Care Consensus No. 8. American College of Obstetricians and Gynecologists. Obstet Gynecol 2019;133:e51–72. Available at: https://oce.ovid.com/article/00006250-201901000-00051/HTML.
5. World Health Organization. Report of a WHO technical consultation on birth spacing. Geneva (Switzerland): WHO Press; 2007. WHO/RHR/07.1 World Health Organization; Available at: http://www.who.int/making_pregnancy_safer/documents/birth_spacing05/en/index.html. Accessed: December 5, 2019.
6. Conde-Agudelo A, Rosas-Bermudez A, Kafury-Goeta A. Birth spacing and risk of adverse perinatal outcomes: a meta-analysis. JAMA 2006;295:1809–23.
7. White K, Teal S, Potter J. Contraception after delivery and short interpregnancy intervals among women in the United States. Obstet Gynecol 2015;125:1471–7.
8. Gemmill A, Lindberg LD. Short interpregnancy intervals in the United States. Obstet Gynecol 2013;122:64–71.
9. Kaplan RM. Shared medical decision making. A new tool for preventive medicine. Am J Prev Med 2004;26(1):81–3.
10. Dehlendorf C, Levy K, Kelley A, et al. Women's preferences for contraceptive counseling and decision-making. Contraception 2013;88:250–6.
11. de Haes H. Dilemmas in patient centeredness and shared decision making: a case for vulnerability. Patient Educ Couns 2006;62:291–8.
12. Dehlendorf C, Grumbach K, Schmittdiel J, et al. Shared decision making in contraceptive counseling. Contraception 2017;95(5):452–5.
13. Uhm S, Shah A, Whie K. Women's preferences for prenatal contraceptive counseling. Contraception 2018;98(4):360.
14. Zapata L, Murtaza S, Whiteman M, et al. Contraceptive counseling and postpartum contraceptive use. Am J Obstet Gynecol 2015;212:171.e1–8.
15. Cwiak C, Gellasch T, Zieman M. Peripartum contraceptive attitudes and practices. Contraception 2004;70:383–6.

16. Stern A. Sterilized in the name of public health: race, immigration, and reproductive control in modern California. Am J Public Health 2005;95:1128–38.

17. Harris L, Wolfe T. Stratified reproduction, family planning care and the double edge of history. Curr Opin Obstet Gynecol 2017;26:539–44.

18. Ross L, Roberts L, Derkas E, et al. Radical reproductive justice. New York: Feminist Press; 2017.

19. Ross L. Understanding Reproductive Justice. SisterSong Women of Color Reproductive Health Collective, May 2006. Available at: https://d3n8a8pro7vhmx. cloudfront.net/rrfp/pages/33/attachments/original/1456425809/Understanding_ RJ_Sistersong.pdf?1456425809. Accessed December 20, 2019.

20. Centers for Disease Control. Update to CDC's U.S. medical eligibility criteria for contraceptive use, 2010: revised recommendations for the use of contraceptive methods during the postpartum period. Available at: https://www.cdc.gov/ mmwr/volumes/65/rr/pdfs/rr6503.pdf. Accessed December 20, 2019.

21. Trussell J. Contraceptive failure in the United States. Contraception 2011;83(5): 397–404.

22. Nuvaring [package insert]. Whitehouse Station (NJ): Merck and Co, Inc; 2001-2018. Available at: http://www.merck.com/product/usa/pi_circulars/n/nuvaring/ nuvaring_pi.pdf. Accessed December 20, 2019.

23. Annovera [package insert]. New York: Manufactured for Population Council; 2018. Available at: www.accessdata.fda.gov/drugsatfda_docs/label/2018/ 209627s000lbl.pdf. Accessed December 20, 2019.

24. Hatcher R, Trussell J, Nelson A, et al. Contraceptive technology. New York: Ardent Media, Inc.; 2007.

25. Rowe P, Farley T, Peregoudov A, et al. Safety and efficacy in parous women of a 52-mg levonorgestrel-medicated intrauterine device: a 7-year randomized comparative study with the TCu380A. Contraception 2016;93(6):498–506.

26. McNicholas C, Swor E, Wan L, et al. Prolonged use of the etonogestrel implant and levonorgestrel intrauterine device–two years beyond FDA-approved duration. Am J Obstet Gynecol 2017;216(6):586.e1–6.

27. World Health Organization. Long-term reversible contraception: twelve years of experience with the TCu380A and TCu220C. Contraception 1997;56(6):341–52.

28. Cohen R, Sheeder J, Arango N, et al. Twelve-month contraceptive continuation and repeat pregnancy among young mothers choosing post-delivery contraceptive implants or postplacental intrauterine devices. Contraception 2016;93: 178–83.

29. Whitaker A, Chen B. Society of Family Planning guidelines: postplacental insertion of intrauterine devices. Contraception 2018;97(1):2–13.

30. Bullock H, Salcedo J. Emergency contraception: do your patients have plan B? Obstet Gynecol Clin North Am 2015;42:699–712.

31. Faculty of Family Planning and Reproductive Health Care Clinical Effectiveness Unit. Contraceptive choices for breastfeeding women. J Fam Plann Reprod Health Care 2004;30:181–9.

32. Sober S, Schreiber C. Postpartum contraception. Clin Obstet Gynecol 2014; 57(4):763–76.

33. Daniels K, Daugherty J, Jones J. Current contraceptive status among women aged 15–44: United States, Department of Health and Human Services 2011–2013. NCHS data brief, CDC 2014:1–8.

34. Zite N, Wuellner S, Gilliam M. Failure to obtain desired postpartum sterilization: risk and predictors. Obstet Gynecol 2005;105:794–9.

35. Seibel-Seamon J, Visintine J, Leiby B, et al. Factors predictive for failure to perform postpartum tubal ligations following vaginal delivery. J Reprod Med 2009;54:160–4.
36. Wolfe K, Wilson M, Hou M, et al. An updated assessment of postpartum sterilization fulfillment after vaginal delivery. Contraception 2017;96(1):41–6.
37. Hahn T, Tucker-Edmonds B, Layman S, et al. A prospective study on the effects of Medicaid regulation and other barriers to obtaining postpartum sterilization. J Midwifery Womens Health 2019;64(2):186–938.
38. Moniz M, Chang T, Heisler M, et al. Inpatient postpartum long-acting reversible contraception and sterilization in the United States, 2008-2013. Obstet Gynecol 2017;129(6):1078–85.
39. Thurman A, Janecek T. One-year follow-up of women with unfulfilled postpartum sterilization requests. Obstet Gynecol 2010;116:1071–7.
40. Arora K, Wilkinson B, Verbus E, et al. Medicaid and fulfillment of desired postpartum sterilization. Contraception 2018;97(6):559–64.
41. Gilliam M, Davis S, Berlin A, et al. A qualitative study of barriers to postpartum sterilization and women's attitudes toward unfulfilled sterilization requests. Contraception 2008;77:44–9.

Diagnosis and Management of Postpartum Pelvic Floor Disorders

Ana Rebecca Meekins, MD*, Nazema Y. Siddiqui, MD, MHS

KEYWORDS

- Postpartum • Pelvic floor disorders • Urinary incontinence • Fecal incontinence
- Pelvic organ prolapse

KEY POINTS

- Urinary incontinence is not uncommon in the postpartum period and in most cases can be managed conservatively.
- Women who sustain an obstetric anal sphincter injury are more likely to have fecal incontinence postpartum and should be evaluated to assess integrity of the anal sphincter complex.
- Pelvic organ prolapse tends to occur later in life, but can develop in the postpartum period and our general recommendation is conservative management for symptomatic women within 1 year of delivery.

POSTPARTUM BLADDER CONTROL

It is well-known that bladder function can change during pregnancy and the postpartum period. The physiology of the lower urinary tract is complex and depends on interactions between the central, peripheral, and autonomic nervous systems (**Fig. 1**). The bladder must be able to appropriately fill and empty. These processes are differentially regulated by the sympathetic and parasympathetic nervous systems, respectively. During filling, bladder volume increases in the setting of sympathetic signaling. Norepinephrine is the primary neurotransmitter of the sympathetic nervous system. Norepinephrine stimulates beta-adrenergic receptors on the bladder to allow for detrusor smooth muscle relaxation. At the same time, norepinephrine stimulates alpha-adrenergic receptors on the urethra to facilitate urethral smooth muscle contraction. In contrast, emptying the bladder is a voluntary act that involves central nervous system signaling through the spinal cord and pelvic nerves to facilitate urethral and pelvic floor muscle relaxation. This is immediately followed by

Department of Obstetrics and Gynecology, Division of Urogynecology, Duke University School of Medicine, 5324 McFarland Drive Suite 310, Durham, NC 27707, USA
* Corresponding author.
E-mail address: Rebecca.Meekins@duke.edu

Obstet Gynecol Clin N Am 47 (2020) 477–486
https://doi.org/10.1016/j.ogc.2020.05.002
0889-8545/20/© 2020 Elsevier Inc. All rights reserved.

obgyn.theclinics.com

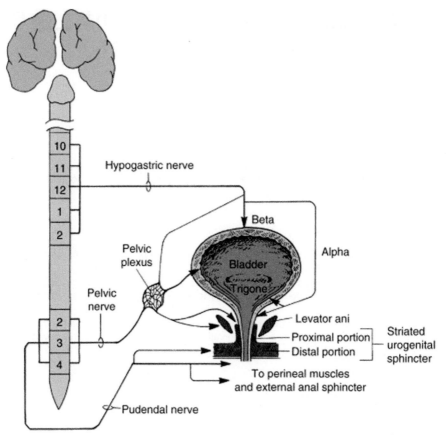

Fig. 1. Peripheral innervation of the female lower urinary tract. (*From* Hale DS, Walters MD. Neurophysiology and Pharmacology of the Lower Urinary Tract. In: Walters MD, Karram MM, editors. Urogynecology and reconstructive pelvic surgery, 4th edition. Philadelphia: Elsevier; 2015; with permission.)

parasympathetic signaling through its primary neurotransmitter, acetylcholine. Acetylcholine signaling stimulates the detrusor muscle to contract and empty the bladder.

Postpartum women may experience a wide array of urinary changes from urinary leakage to incomplete emptying. When a postpartum patient presents with changes in bladder function there are a few broad categories to consider in approaching diagnosis and treatment:

1. Urinary tract infection (UTI);
2. Bladder overdistention injury; and
3. Altered muscular control of the pelvic floor.

UTI results in bladder inflammation with subsequent symptoms of frequency, urgency, pain, and/or incontinence. Assessing for pyuria (increased white blood cells) on urinalysis is the first step in evaluating for UTI. In the postpartum setting, lochia may confound urinalysis results when voided urine samples are used. Unless a catheterized sample is obtained, subsequent urine culture testing is recommended in the setting of pyuria to confirm the diagnosis of UTI and avoid inappropriate use of antibiotics. During labor or the postpartum period, if the patient has a large volume of urine in the bladder, a bladder overdistension injury could occur. If epidural or spinal anesthesia is used, large urine volumes may go unrecognized because the patient will lack sensations of bladder filling. Even after anesthesia is discontinued, there may be a temporal delay of many hours until return of full bladder sensation. Bladder overdistention injuries are typically self-limited and resolve within a few weeks. However, supportive care may be needed during that time, as well as education on frequent voiding to avoid repeat episodes of overdistention. Finally, a postpartum patient may exhibit changes in bladder function owing to alterations in the musculature of the pelvic floor. This is more common after vaginal or operative delivery, where pelvic floor laxity or injury may result in urgency, frequency, or incontinence. However, regardless of the mode of delivery, some women also develop increased pelvic muscle tone and spasm, which can result in urinary hesitancy or difficulty voiding. In this section, we focus on the presentation, diagnosis, and treatment of the most common bladder complaint in postpartum women, namely, urinary incontinence.

Stress Urinary Incontinence

Women may present to the clinic during and after pregnancy with complaints of leaking urine with coughing, laughing, sneezing, or activity. This presentation is classic for stress urinary incontinence (SUI). SUI results from a laxity in urethral support and subsequent inability of the urethra to remain closed during events that cause increased intra-abdominal pressure. SUI can be easily confirmed during pelvic examination by asking the patient to cough or Valsalva with a full bladder. If the provider observes urine leaking from the urethra during an office cough/Valsalva stress test, the diagnosis of SUI is confirmed. Based on the Value of Urodynamic Evaluation study, in women with uncomplicated SUI without significant prolapse or urinary urgency, if SUI is demonstrated on examination, additional urodynamic testing is not necessary before treatment.[1]

If SUI is observed on examination, treatment may be facilitated by assessing the pelvic floor muscle strength. This assessment can be done during digital vaginal examination while asking the patient to squeeze her pelvic floor, also known as a Kegel contraction. Patients with good proprioception and ability to contract their pelvic floor are candidates for home pelvic floor exercises. Both the American Urogynecologic Society and the International Urogynecological Association have patient resources available to guide home exercises: https://www.augs.org/assets/2/6/Bladder_Training.pdf; https://thepelvicfloorsociety.co.uk/budcms/includes/kcfinder/upload/files/eng_pfe.pdf. Notably, if the patient lacks proprioception or is unable to generate a moderate squeeze on pelvic floor contraction, it is unlikely they will make progress without guided exercises. For these patients, or for those who have tried home exercises without significant improvement in SUI, referral to pelvic floor physical therapy (PFPT) is a logical next step in management. Certified women's health physical therapists can more thoroughly evaluate the pelvic floor, create a personalized exercise plan, and monitor progress over time. Although the postpartum period is busy and additional appointments may not be desired, patient satisfaction with PFPT is quite high, and depending on their level of bother, some women may prefer this option.[2]

Anti-incontinence devices are also an option for conservative management of SUI. These devices are placed within the vagina and provide urethral support. There are over-the-counter disposable tampon-like devices, such as Impressa, that patients can trial at home. Alternatively, an incontinence pessary can be fitted in the office. Patients can typically manage these on their own after teaching on proper placement and removal.

Although not a classic treatment device for SUI, wearable technology has been applied to protective garments for symptom management. For women with mild to moderate leakage, there are now multiple options of absorbent, leak-proof, and odor-resistant underwear that can be used instead of pads or panty liners. These products are extensions of absorbent underwear designed for menstruation and are also machine washable. Knowledge of these products can further aid with symptom control while women are pursuing conservative management.

If conservative measures are insufficient to improve quality of life, the next step is referral to a specialist in female pelvic medicine and reconstructive surgery for additional evaluation and management. This evaluation could include a discussion of surgical options such as a midurethral sling. Of note, we do not recommend proceeding with anti-incontinence surgery in patients who have not yet completed child bearing.

Urgency Urinary Incontinence

Although more common after 40 years of age, involuntary urinary leakage associated with urgency can occur in women of all ages, and is called urgency urinary incontinence. Urgency urinary incontinence occurs in a subset of women with an overactive bladder (OAB), which is a syndrome defined by the International Continence Society as "symptoms of urinary urgency, usually accompanied by frequency and nocturia, with or without urgency urinary incontinence, in the absence of urinary tract infection or other obvious pathology."[3]

OAB is typically diagnosed based on history and a screening urinalysis. Important components of the history that can be helpful include the interval of time between voids, triggers for urinary leakage, degree of leakage (pads used per day), presence of nighttime symptoms, and level of bother. In addition, reviewing current medications, recent changes in medication, and fluid intake can be helpful. If the patient is not able to provide a clear picture of their bladder habits, we recommend completing a 3-day bladder diary. The American Urogynecologic Society provides a sample bladder diary template online: https://www.voicesforpfd.org/assets/2/6/Voiding_Diary.pdf.

Diagnosis rarely requires additional urologic testing. That being said, urodynamic testing can be helpful if there is concern for a neurologic component to OAB symptoms. Thus, in postpartum women, urodynamic testing may be considered if there are new-onset urinary symptoms and concern for pelvic nerve injury (eg, after a prolonged second stage of labor or operative vaginal delivery). In addition, urodynamic testing may also be considered in women with prolonged voiding difficulties or high postvoid residuals after suspected bladder overdistention injury. In both of these instances, urodynamic testing could help with diagnosis, and determining prognosis.

The first-line treatment for women with uncomplicated OAB includes many conservative measures. First of all, women should be counseled on behavioral changes, such as using timed voids (ie, emptying the bladder every 2–3 hours), limiting fluid intake such that they drink when thirsty, and avoiding bladder irritants such as ingested artificial sweeteners, acidic or alcoholic beverages, and caffeine.

First-line therapy also includes pelvic floor strengthening. Data regarding this practice are not conclusive, but the risk is minimal and therefore it is reasonable to counsel patients on this option.[4] Contraction of the pelvic floor leads to an inhibitory reflex via the spinal pathway that causes bladder relaxation. For example, women who have control of their pelvic floor muscles can be instructed to perform pelvic muscle contractions either when the urge starts or just before an event that typically triggers an urge (ie, pulling the car into the driveway). This muscle contraction leads to increased bladder relaxation and provides additional time to reach a restroom without leaking. Some women may benefit from referral to PFPT. This strategy is especially helpful for women who lack proprioception or have less control over their pelvic floor muscles, and therefore would benefit from direct feedback with the use of biofeedback.

Second-line therapy for OAB involves the use of medications. There are 2 overarching classes of medications for OAB that target different nerve receptors:

1. Anticholinergics; and
2. Beta-agonists.

There are several anticholinergic medications available that exert their effects by blocking acetylcholine from binding to muscarinic nerve receptors in the bladder. When acetylcholine is unable to effectively stimulate the bladder, there is less bladder contraction and therefore less urgency. Many studies have looked at the effectiveness of anticholinergic medications and collectively have only shown a modest effect over placebo in decreasing leakage episodes and number of voids per day.[5] Additionally, these medications are not tissue specific and have well-known side effects including dry mouth, dry eye, constipation, and in some cases cognitive changes. One systematic review found that 1% to 6% of patients enrolled in randomized trials discontinued medications owing to adverse effects, whereas a mixed-methods study in a more generalizable population found that approximately 30% of women discontinued medications owing to adverse events or intolerability.[6,7] In the postpartum population, one must also consider compatibility with breastfeeding. There is very limited information on the safety of these medications in lactating women. Given the known systemic anticholinergic effects, lactating postpartum women may also need to monitor for a reduction in milk production (https://toxnet.nlm.nih.gov/cgi-bin/sis/search2).

Beta 3-adrenergic receptor agonists constitute another class of medications that are used to treat OAB. Beta agonists enhance sympathetic nerve signaling to increase detrusor muscle relaxation. Although other alternatives may be available in the future, currently mirabegron is the only available drug in this class. The efficacy of mirabegron is similar to anticholinergic medications, although the adverse event profile is different.[8] Mirabegron does not have anticholinergic side effects, but instead can cause an increase in blood pressure. Thus, this drug should not be used in patients with uncontrolled hypertension. There are no data regarding the safety of mirabegron in lactating women.

It is reasonable to refer to female pelvic medicine and reconstructive surgery at any time during the evaluation or management of a patient with OAB. However, we strongly recommend referral in patients where additional testing, such as urodynamics, would be warranted, or in instances where first- and second-line therapies have failed.

It should be noted that the pelvic floor is dynamic after pregnancy and delivery. Even without intervention, many women may experience improvements in urinary symptoms over the course of weeks to months. There are limited data on the progression of urinary incontinence symptoms in women over time. A recent study by Hagan and colleagues[9] did not specifically address postpartum women but looked at the natural history of urinary incontinence in a cohort of women over 10 years. They found that younger women were more likely to have improvement or complete remission of symptoms as compared with older women. Additionally, women with less severe symptoms were also more likely to report improvement over time.

POSTPARTUM BOWEL CONTROL

Postpartum women can experience significant short- and long-term changes in bowel function after pregnancy. Women at highest risk for bowel control issues are those who sustain obstetric anal sphincter injuries (OASIS), which includes third- and fourth-degree perineal lacerations.

The Childbirth and Pelvic Symptom Study found that 26% of women with OASIS had fecal incontinence at 6 weeks postpartum. By 6 months after delivery, this prevalence only dropped to 17%, as compared with 7% to 8% of those who had cesarean delivery or vaginal delivery without OASIS.[10] Long-term outcomes were assessed as part of the large prospective Mothers' Outcomes After Delivery study, which found that OASIS is significantly associated with fecal incontinence as long as 5 to 10 years postpartum.[11] This association was found to be persistent at 15 to 23 years after delivery in a large prospective Scandinavian study.[12] Although a significant number of women with OASIS continue to have fecal incontinence, we know that the majority of women who are initially symptomatic will experience resolution of symptoms over the first 3 years postpartum.[13] Notably, the most important risk factor for having continued bowel control issues was the presence of a persistent anal sphincter defect, highlighting the importance of an adequate primary repair if OASIS occurs. Women who experience OASIS are candidates for early postpartum follow-up within the first 2 to 4 weeks to evaluate for appropriate healing or the presence of ongoing symptoms that might suggest a persistent defect. Furthermore, women who experience perineal injury after childbirth, and especially those with injury to the anal sphincter, should be educated on what might be considered inappropriate perineal pain and/or drainage in the early weeks after childbirth, and encouraged to present for evaluation if these symptoms occur.

Risk factors for OASIS are well-known and include, but are not limited to, maternal age, nulliparity, body mass index, race and ethnicity, prior OASIS, prior cesarean section, fetal macrosomia, obstetric factors such as shoulder dystocia and fetal position, operative vaginal delivery (including forceps and vacuum), episiotomy, and duration of second stage of labor.[14–16] Many of these risk factors are not modifiable and currently there is limited ability to counsel women on their individual risk of OASIS at the time of delivery. There are some evidence-based preventative strategies, including antepartum perineal massage and warm compresses to the perineum during the second stage of labor, but it is unclear how often these interventions are being used.[17]

When a patient presents during the postpartum period with fecal incontinence, the evaluation should focus on determining if an anal sphincter defect is present. This factor can be assessed on physical examination by performing a careful external genital and digital rectal examination. First, evaluate the perineal body. After a large perineal laceration, if the muscles of the perineal body or external anal sphincter are not reapproximated, the patient may have a very short, thin perineal body with minimal tissue separating the posterior vagina and anal opening. A digital rectal examination will help in assessing perineal body bulk while also providing information regarding anal sphincter tone and ability for the patient to generate an anal sphincter contraction. When assessing tone and squeeze pressures, the examiner should focus on whether or not the squeeze is circumferential or if a particular area is weak.

If a persistent anal sphincter defect is suspected, it is critical to proceed with further evaluation. Generally, functional and neuromuscular outcomes improve with early sphincter repair. Therefore, the next step would be to refer to a specialist who can evaluate and manage sphincter trauma. In many regions, this professional is a specialist in female pelvic medicine and reconstructive surgery, although in some centers, colorectal surgeons may offer this care. During evaluation, endoanal ultrasound examination is helpful in identifying the extent and location of both internal and external anal sphincter defects, which is useful in guiding surgical planning.

Treatment for a confirmed symptomatic anal sphincter defect includes anal sphinc-teroplasty. Based on data from a large systematic review, success rates decrease over time after sphincteroplasty, but the majority of women remain satisfied with their outcome. It is important to understand that the outcomes of anal sphincteroplasty are worse when performed more than 10 years after initial trauma, in postmenopausal women where muscle atrophy has occurred, and if there is evidence of pudendal neu-ropathy.[18] In line with Practice Bulletin recommendations from the American College of Obstetrics and Gynecology, after childbirth with an anal sphincter injury, women should be counseled that the risk of recurrence with a future vaginal delivery is low but should also be given the option of elective cesarean section for subsequent deliv-eries with appropriate discussion of surgical risks.[19] If anal sphincteroplasty is required to correct defects in the anal sphincter and the woman desires future child-bearing, strong consideration should be given to cesarean delivery in subsequent pregnancies.

If a postpartum patient has symptoms of fecal incontinence without evidence of anal sphincter defect, treatment should focus on regulating bowel habits and optimizing pelvic floor muscle control. In these patients, we recommend first normalizing bowel consistency and frequency using fiber supplementation and dietary changes as needed. Referral to PFPT is also an appropriate next step for these patients. PFPT can assist with pelvic floor strengthening, relaxation and coordination by using manual internal work and biofeedback through vaginal and transanal routes, as appropriate. If a patient has tried and failed conservative management for fecal incontinence, we recommend referral to a specialist for further evaluation and consideration of advanced therapies, such as sacral neuromodulation.[20,21]

POSTPARTUM PELVIC ORGAN SUPPORT AND RISK OF PROLAPSE

We know from recent data that the incidence of pelvic organ prolapse (POP) 15 years after first vaginal delivery is significant.[22] Furthermore, these data also demonstrate that the incidence of POP is significantly higher among those with a history of vaginal delivery as compared with those who had undergone cesarean delivery.[22] It is not entirely clear who is at greatest risk of developing prolapse later in life, but we are beginning to have an improved understanding of the obstetric risk factors that contribute to POP. Importantly, we now know that women who sustain levator muscle avulsion, which is most likely to occur during a forceps-assisted delivery, are more likely to develop POP beyond the hymen.[23]

Although it is important to understand these long-term impacts of childbirth on pel-vic organ support, we focus here on how to approach the patient who presents in the postpartum or intrapartum period with prolapse. There is a paucity of data regarding prolapse outcomes in this population and much of this section is based on our expert opinion. Importantly, it is thought that it takes a woman's body several months to re-turn to a normal physiologic state after pregnancy. It can therefore be assumed that vaginal tissue, like the rest of the body, is likely undergoing healing and tissue remod-eling for several months postpartum. Additionally, although breastfeeding has not been associated with development of pelvic floor disorders 1 to 2 decades after a woman's first vaginal delivery, it is reasonable to assume that the lack of estrogen dur-ing lactation further influences the return of normal vaginal structure and function in the postpartum period.[24] With those considerations in mind, it is our general recommen-dation that women with symptomatic prolapse delay any surgical intervention until at least 12 months postpartum. This strategy will allow ample time for any potential tissue remodeling to occur that could change or improve vaginal support. Additionally, we do not recommend surgical interventions for POP until a woman has completed child-bearing. Nonsurgical treatment options may be offered including home pelvic floor exercises or referral to PFPT for mild to moderate prolapse, or the use of a pessary in more advanced symptomatic prolapse.

POSTPARTUM SEXUAL DYSFUNCTION

It is well-known that childbirth impacts sexual function. These changes may lead to a variety of adverse physical, psychological, and social effects, and may decrease quality of life. In 1 study of more than 300 women, 64% reported sexual dysfunction and 70% reported sexual dissatisfaction during the first 12 months postpartum.[25] In this study, risk factors identified for sexual dysfunction included late return to intercourse after delivery (≥9 weeks), primiparity, and depression, among others.[25,26] Vaginal delivery leads to anatomic and functional changes in the pelvic floor muscles, which might be responsible for some of women's complaints about sexual problems during the postpartum period.[27] Perineal pain and dyspareunia are common experiences for postnatal women. Women who sustain an injury to the anal sphincter are more likely to experience longer periods of perineal pain and dyspareunia. These women are also more likely to report a decrease in the frequency of sexual intercourse and reduced sexual desire. Hormonal effects associated with breastfeeding seem to be associated with vaginal dryness and loss of libido.[28] Notably, women who undergo a cesarean section have been found to have less sexual dysfunction in the short term compared with women who underwent a vaginal delivery, but this difference does not persist past 6 months postpartum.[29]

Clinicians should be prepared to address concerns regarding sexual function after childbirth in the postpartum period. Follow-up should be provided for those women who experience perineal pain and dyspareunia when they resume sexual activity. Given that levator spasm can result from prolonged perineal pain, early referral to PFPT can be beneficial to prevent further pelvic floor dysfunction in this setting.

SUMMARY

Pelvic floor disorders affect quality of life in the postpartum period and beyond. Urinary incontinence can greatly impact quality of life. Obstetricians should be familiar with the evaluation and initial management of urinary incontinence to help women cope with this bothersome and common problem. POP can occur in the short term after childbirth; surgical intervention is generally delayed until completion of childbearing and at least 12 months after delivery. Fecal incontinence as a result of injury to the pelvic floor might be under-reported by the woman owing to embarrassment and delayed follow-up postpartum. It is important to remember that women who experience perineal injury, and especially those with an anal sphincter injury, are candidates for early postpartum follow-up within the first 2 to 4 weeks to evaluate healing and return to function. Sexual dysfunction is also common in the postpartum period, and may require additional follow-up. For many postpartum pelvic floor disorders, PFPT can be extremely helpful for initial management. Women at risk for pelvic floor disorders after childbirth should be counseled and encouraged to seek early follow-up in the postpartum period so that symptoms may be appropriately evaluated, treated, and referred in a timely manner if conservative treatment options fail to resolve symptoms.

DISCLOSURE

The authors have nothing to disclose.

REFERENCES

1. Nager CW, Brubaker L, Litman HJ, et al. A randomized trial of urodyanmic testing before stress-incontinence surgery. N Engl J Med 2012;366(21):1987–97.
2. Richter HE, Burgio KL, Brubaker L, et al. Continence pessary compared with behavioral therapy or combined therapy for stress incontinence: a randomized controlled trial. Obstet Gynecol 2010;115(3):609–17.
3. Haylen BT, de Ridder D, Freeman RM, et al. An International Urogynecological Association (IUGA)/International Continence Society (ICS) joint report on the terminology for female pelvic floor dysfunction. Neurourol Urodyn 2010;29(1):4–20.
4. Monteiro S, Riccetto C, Araújo A, et al. Efficacy of pelvic floor muscle training in women with overactive bladder syndrome: a systematic review. Int Urogynecol J 2018;29(11):1565–73.
5. Reynolds WS, McPheeters M, Blume J, et al. Comparative effectiveness of anticholinergic therapy for overactive bladder in women: a systematic review and meta-analysis. Obstet Gynecol 2015;125(6):1423–32.
6. Shamliyan T, Wyman JF, Ramakrishnan R, et al. Benefits and harms of pharmacologic treatment for urinary incontinence in women: a systematic review. Ann Intern Med 2012;156(12):861–74. W301-10.
7. Diokno AC, Sand PK, Macdiarmid S, et al. Perceptions and behaviours of women with bladder control problems. Fam Pract 2006;23(5):568–77.
8. Sebastianelli A, Russo GI, Kaplan SA, et al. Systematic review and meta-analysis on the efficacy and tolerability of mirabegron for the treatment of storage lower urinary tract symptoms/overactive bladder: comparison with placebo and tolterodine. Int J Urol 2018;25(3):196–205.
9. Hagan KA, Erekson E, Austin A, et al. A prospective study of the natural history of urinary incontinence in women. Am J Obstet Gynecol 2018;218(5):502.e1-8.
10. Borello-France D, Burgio KL, Richter HE, et al. Fecal and urinary incontinence in primiparous women. Obstet Gynecol 2006;108(4):863–72.
11. Evers EC, Blomquist JL, McDermott KC, et al. Obstetrical anal sphincter laceration and anal incontinence 5-10 years after childbirth. Am J Obstet Gynecol 2012; 207(5):425.e1-6.
12. Halle TK, Salvesen KÅ, Volløyhaug I. Obstetric anal sphincter injury and incontinence 15-23 years after vaginal delivery. Acta Obstet Gynecol Scand 2016;95(8): 941–7.
13. Reid AJ, Beggs AD, Sultan AH, et al. Outcome of repair of obstetric anal sphincter injuries after three years. Int J Gynaecol Obstet 2014;127(1):47–50.
14. Lowder JL, Burrows LJ, Krohn MA, et al. Risk factors for primary and subsequent anal sphincter lacerations: a comparison of cohorts by parity and prior mode of delivery. Am J Obstet Gynecol 2007;196(4):344.e1-5.
15. Marschalek ML, Worda C, Kuessel L, et al. Risk and protective factors for obstetric anal sphincter injuries: a retrospective nationwide study. Birth 2018;45(4): 409–15.
16. Davies-Tuck M, Biro MA, Mockler J, et al. Maternal Asian ethnicity and the risk of anal sphincter injury. Acta Obstet Gynecol Scand 2015;94(3):308–15.
17. Aasheim V, Nilsen AB, Lukasse M, et al. Perineal techniques during the second stage of labour for reducing perineal trauma. Cochrane Database Syst Rev 2011;(12):CD006672.
18. Glasgow SC, Lowry AC. Long-term outcomes of anal sphincter repair for fecal incontinence: a systematic review. Dis Colon Rectum 2012;55(4):482–90.

19. Committee on Practice Bulletins-Obstetrics. ACOG practice Bulletin No. 198: prevention and management of obstetric lacerations at vaginal delivery. Obstet Gynecol 2018;132(3):e87–102.

20. Thaha MA, Abukar AA, Thin NN, et al. Sacral nerve stimulation for faecal incontinence and constipation in adults. Cochrane Database Syst Rev 2015;(8):CD004464.

21. Rydningen MB, Dehli T, Wilsgaard T, et al. Sacral neuromodulation for faecal incontinence following obstetric sphincter injury - outcome of percutaneous nerve evaluation. Colorectal Dis 2017;19(3):274–82.

22. Blomquist JL, Muñoz A, Carroll M, et al. Association of delivery mode with pelvic floor disorders after childbirth. JAMA 2018;320(23):2438–47.

23. Handa VL, Blomquist JL, Roem J, et al. Pelvic floor disorders after obstetric avulsion of the levator ani muscle. Female Pelvic Med Reconstr Surg 2019;25(1):3–7.

24. Lovejoy DA, Roem JL, Blomquist JL, et al. Breastfeeding and pelvic floor disorders one to two decades after vaginal delivery. Am J Obstet Gynecol 2019; 221(4):333.e1-8.

25. Sayasneh A, Pandeva I. Postpartum sexual dysfunction: a literature review of risk factors and role of mode of delivery. British Journal of Medical Practitioners 2010; 3(2):316–20.

26. Khajehei M, Doherty M, Tilley PJM, et al. Prevalence and risk factors of sexual dysfunction in postpartum Australian women. J Sex Med 2015;12:1415–26.

27. Shahraki Z, Tanha FD, Ghajarzadeh M. Depression, sexual dysfunction and sexual quality of life in women with infertility. BMC Womens Health 2018;18(1):92.

28. Barrett G, Pendry E, Peacock J, et al. Women's sexual health after childbirth. BJOG 2000;107(2):186–95.

29. Barrett G, Peacock J, Victor CR, et al. Cesarean section and postnatal sexual health. Birth 2005;32(4):306–11.

Pregnancy Complications, Cardiovascular Risk Factors, and Future Heart Disease

Haywood L. Brown, MD[a],*, Graeme N. Smith, MD, PhD[b]

KEYWORDS

- Heart disease mortality • Women • Pregnancy complications • Cardiovascular risk
- Pregnancy • Inflammatory phenotype • Cardiovascular disease
- Lifestyle modification

KEY POINTS

- Women with high parity and pregnancy complications of preeclampsia, gestational diabetes, and low birth weight are at increased risk for adult cardiovascular morbidity and mortality.
- Assessment of women at risk for cardiovascular disease should begin in the postpartum period.
- Breastfeeding may provide some protection against development of cardiovascular disease.
- Education of women and providers is essential to prevention of cardiovascular morbidity and mortality.
- Women with pregnancy complications are uniquely at risk and should have periodic screening, and institute lifestyle modifications to decrease risk for cardiovascular disease mortality.

INTRODUCTION

Heart disease is the leading cause of mortality for women. In 2013, 1 (35%) in 3 deaths in women worldwide were from cardiovascular disease (CVD).[1,2] The population adjusted risk of CVD mortality is greater for women than men at 20.9% versus 14.9%, respectively.[3] Although the American Heart Association (AHA) states the risk for death from cardiovascular disease has decreased significantly for both women and men since 2000, the mortality for women was higher than that for men since the 1980s and the decline much slower.[1,4] Based on recent data, the gender gap

[a] Department of Obstetrics and Gynecology, Diversity, Morsani College of Medicine, University of South Florida, 13101 Bruce B. Downs Drive, MDC- 3rd Floor, Tampa, FL 33612, USA; [b] Obstetrics & Gynecology, Department of Obstetrics & Gynecology, Queen's University, 76 Stuart Street, Kingston, Ontario K7L 2V7, Canada
* Corresponding author.
E-mail address: haywoodb@usf.edu

Obstet Gynecol Clin N Am 47 (2020) 487–495
https://doi.org/10.1016/j.ogc.2020.04.009
0889-8545/20/Crown Copyright © 2020 Published by Elsevier Inc. All rights reserved.

obgyn.theclinics.com

remains, with the rate of death per 100,000 populations for women at 209 per 100,000 compared with 129.6 per 100,000 in 2017; a slight decline from 2010 for both genders.[1,4]

Unfortunately, only 45% of women and fewer than half of all primary care physicians identify heart disease as the leading cause for death in women or CVD as the top concern for adult women's health despite efforts to raise nationwide awareness.[5]

Over the past decade, there has been growing evidence that women with a history of certain common pregnancy complications confer an increased risk for later development of CVD.[6–11] These include pregnancy conditions such as preeclampsia, gestational diabetes, and low birth weight due to preterm delivery or fetal growth restriction (**Box 1**).

Pregnancy has been referred to as a CVD "physiologic stress test"; women who develop these pregnancy complications are more likely to be identified with underlying, often undiagnosed, cardiovascular risk factors and are at higher risk CVD.[12] The physiologic changes of pregnancy indicate that 20% to 30% have at least 1 traditional or pregnancy-related risk factor that is a predictor for later development of CVD.[13,14]

Previous studies suggest a relationship with increased parity and CVD. In a study from 24 British towns of 4286 women and 4252 men aged 60 to 79 years with at least 2 children, each additional child increased the age-adjusted odds of coronary heart disease (CHD) by 30% (odds ratio, 1.30; 95% confidence interval [CI] 1.17–1.44) for women and by 12% for men (odds ratio [OR] 1.12; 95% confidence interval, 1.02–1.22). Adjustment for obesity and metabolic risk factors attenuated the associations between greater number of children and CHD in both sexes, although in women some association remained.[15] In a more recent study composed of a diverse U.S. cohort, a history of 5+ live births was associated with CVD risk, specifically, myocardial infarction, independent of breastfeeding.

Having a prior pregnancy and no live birth is associated with greater CVD and heart failure risk.[16] The theory behind this increase risk for CVD related to parity is through the cardiometabolic changes of the cumulative number of pregnancies, including weight gain, increased waist circumference, hyperlipidemia, and subclinical atherosclerosis. Women with higher parity had a higher body mass index (BMI), lower

---

Box 1
Female-specific and pregnancy-related risk factors for cardiovascular disease

Pregnancy Complications

Hypertensive disorders
  Gestational hypertension
  Preeclampsia
  Eclampsia

Gestational diabetes mellitus

Preterm delivery
  Less than 37 completed weeks gestation

Low birth weight for gestational age (fetal growth restriction)
  Less than 10th percentile birthweight for gestational age

Female-Specific Risk Factors

Polycystic ovary syndrome
  Insulin resistance

Functional hypothalamic amenorrhea

high-density lipoprotein cholesterol, higher triglycerides, and higher low-density lipo-protein cholesterol at baseline than women with fewer births.[17] Other pregnancy-related changes are likely also a factor. These include increased left ventricular mass and systolic volume.[18]

HYPERTENSIVE DISORDERS

Preeclampsia is one of the most common complications of pregnancy, occurring in 3% to 5% of all pregnancies. Preeclampsia is a leading cause of maternal and peri-natal morbidity and maternal mortality. The condition is characterized by hypertension and proteinuria after 20 weeks' gestation. Factors that increase the risk for develop-ment of preeclampsia include obesity, diabetes and preexisting hypertension, advanced reproductive age, and primiparity. The physiologic and anatomic changes of preeclampsia suggest that it is a cardiovascular condition that involves vascular dysfunction, inflammation ,and hypercoagulability.[19]

Long-term complications of women with a history of preeclampsia/eclampsia include chronic hypertension, type 2 diabetes, metabolic syndrome, coronary artery disease, cerebral vascular disease, and end-stage renal disease. Evidence suggests that these acute cardiovascular changes of preeclampsia increase the risk for later development of CVD.[20–24] A meta-analysis of 3.5 million women found that a history of preeclampsia is associated with a significant lifetime risk of stroke, ischemic heart disease, hypertension, and venous thromboembolism.[20] Another study of 2.3 million women found that those with a history of preeclampsia had approximately a twofold risk for early cardiac, cerebral vascular, peripheral vascular disease, and cardiovascu-lar mortality than those without preeclampsia.[25] PREVFEM, a large retrospective study of women with preeclampsia before term conferred a 3.59 times higher risk of hyper-tension before age 40 years compared with an age-matched reference group with an uncomplicated pregnancy.[26] Although the mechanism for the association between preeclampsia and later development of CVD has not been established, there is a strong association with significant vascular endothelial dysfunction and preeclampsia.[27]

GESTATIONAL DIABETES

Gestational diabetes mellitus (GDM), glucose intolerance, occurs in 5% to 10% of pregnancies. Significant risk factors for GDM include obesity and family history of type 2 diabetes in first-degree relatives. GDM increases the risk for the development of type 2 diabetes and CVD.[27,28,29] Ethnicity plays a role in onset of type 2 diabetes in women with GDM. For example, Latin American women with GDM have an earlier pro-gression to type 2 DM compared with white and non-Hispanic black women. Kjos and colleagues[28] reported a 47% cumulative incidence rate for Latin American women with GDM to develop non–insulin dependent diabetes by 5 years after the index preg-nancy. In a recent study of women screened for DM 4 to 12 weeks postpartum from the index pregnancy with GDM, those with earlier gestational age onset of GDM, higher fasting blood glucose, and managed with medication were more likely to develop type 2 DM.[30] A large database analysis of women with GDM showed a signif-icantly higher risk of CVD, including angina pectoris, myocardial infarction, and hyper-tension, over a follow-up period of 7 years postpartum.[27] Women with a history of GDM develop subclinical atherosclerosis,[31] an increased risk of cardiac dysfunc-tion,[32] increased markers of endothelial dysfunction,[33] and metabolic syndrome.[34] A large population-based study in Ontario, Canada, looked at long-term health outcomes after GDM and demonstrated a higher risk for myocardial infarction, coronary bypass, coronary angioplasty, stroke, and carotid endarterectomy.[34]

It is important to evaluate risk for development of CVD in women with GDM. This must begin with screening 4 to 12 weeks postpartum for type 2 diabetes with a 75-g oral glucose tolerance test (OGTT) according to the American College of Obstetricians and Gynecologists (ACOG)[35] or between 6 weeks and 6 months postpartum and an HgA1c every 2 years according to Diabetes Canada[36] in women with GDM and follow-up based on established criteria. Follow-up of these women and the use of established biochemical and hemodynamic markers for cardiovascular morbidity might lead to a decreased risk and severity of cardiovascular events.

PRETERM AND LOW BIRTH WEIGHT

Preterm birth is defined as a birth less than 37 completed weeks' gestation, and occurs in 6% to 12% of all deliveries worldwide. Low birth weight is defined as a newborn weight less than 2500 g at term or less than 5% for gestational age. There is an accumulated body of evidence that suggests idiopathic preterm labor and resultant preterm birth is the result of an upregulation of inflammatory pathway. It is well known that inflammation is an independent predictor of coronary artery disease. Several studies have demonstrated a significant association with preterm delivery and cerebral vascular stoke later in life.[37–42] The hazard ratio for later development of CVD for those women with a preterm birth ranges from 1.3 to 2.6 compared with term births.[38–43] The inflammatory phenotype leading to preterm birth may be the link for those women with preterm birth being at greater risk for CVD. Spontaneous preterm birth doubles the risk of CVD compared with those women with a term birth.[44] A large-scale study tracking mothers' subsequent admissions and deaths over 15 to 19 years indicates an intergenerational influence on birthweight that provides a correlation between the birthweights of parents and their offspring and the associated risk of mortality from CVD.[41] The coincidence of fetal growth restriction and prematurity increased risk for CVD later in life.

There is some evidence that breastfeeding and the duration of breastfeeding has maternal metabolic benefits, including a lower incidence of the metabolic syndrome and provides some protection against CVD.[45] Schwarz and colleagues[46] examined the effect of lactation on CVD risk in 139,681 postmenopausal women in the Women's Preventative Service Initiative (WPSI). There was a dose response relationship; women who had a lifetime history of breastfeeding of more than 12 months were less likely to have hypertension (OR 0.88, $P < .001$), diabetes (OR 0.80, $P < .001$), hyperlipidemia (OR .81, $P < .001$), or CVD (OR 0.91, $P < .001$) compared with women who never breastfed.[46] This was significant despite the confounder of obesity. In another study of 2540 women with CHD who had breastfed for a lifetime total of 2 years or longer, 37% had a lower risk of CHD (95% CI 23%–49%; $P < .001$), adjusting for age, parity, and stillbirth history. This study was also adjusted for early adult adiposity, parental history, and lifestyle factors and even with those confounders the risk reduction was 23% lower for CVD compared with women who never breastfeed.[47] An area for future research is to evaluate the breastfeeding impact on CVD for those with pregnancy complications, preeclampsia, preterm birth, and low birthweight on the later development of CVD.

POSTPARTUM SCREENING

As stated, CVD is the leading cause of premature death for women, and women's cardiovascular health suffers because of male-dominated screening and diagnostic tests and treatments. Women's cardiovascular health has been identified as a key national priority in many countries, which should be addressed through improved awareness, screening, prevention, and intervention, and reducing care inequities for women in general and younger women in particular. Given the costs of treating CVD, novel and innovative ways to identify who should undergo cardiovascular risk (CVR) screening are critical to achieve these goals. For most women, pregnancy and the postpartum period provide a window of opportunity for screening and implementing intervention and therapeutic strategies to improve long-term health and prevent CVD. Postpartum CVR screening, counseling, and lifestyle intervention is now widely considered standard of care following the identified pregnancy complications.[11]

Various publications recommend initiating CVR screening within the first year postpartum, typically between 3 and 6 months. This would take the form of a complete history (including first-degree family history of CVD and CVRs), physical examination (ie, blood pressure, waist circumference, BMI) and biochemical testing (lipid profile, fasting glucose or 75-g OGTT for women with GDM, high-sensitivity C-reactive protein, and urine albumin:creatinine ratio) and counseling about lifestyle modification including physical activity and dietary changes, especially cholesterol and salt reduction. Even small changes in lifestyle can reduce CVR; regular moderate-intensity physical activity and even small amounts of weight loss can have a beneficial effect on lipids and cholesterol.

Postpartum screening and counseling also affords the opportunity for preconception counseling. Going in to the next pregnancy without achieving prepregnancy BMI increases the risks for complications in pregnancy as well as increasing the risk of obesity in the longer term. It is also an opportunity to discuss the importance of earlier screening for GDM (if applicable), initiation of low-dose aspirin for reducing the risk of preeclampsia, and interventions for women with a high risk for recurrent preterm delivery for those with history of idiopathic preterm labor or preterm premature rupture of membranes.

The postpartum visit is the initial step to educate women and counsel them on the importance of optimizing current health and adhering to guidelines for ongoing care. For example, the AHA recommends that all adults $\geq$20 years of age have a cholesterol and other traditional risk factors checked every 4 to 6 years and for those with an elevated lipid profile receive dietary and if appropriate medication to improve the lipid profile. The AHA also recommends that blood pressure (BP) be screened during regular health care visits at least every 2 years for anyone $\geq$20 years of age and for those $\geq$40 years that screening of BP should be annually.[48] As pregnancy after age 40 years has become more common and resultant risk of pregnancy complications for women older than 40 higher, adherence to this recommendation for annual BP follow-up for these women is even more significant. Finally, counseling should occur on the significance of achieving a healthier adult weight and the impact of excessive weight gain during pregnancy and adult weight retention after childbearing have on the later development of diabetes and thereby CVD risk. At postpartum follow-up, women should be encouraged to access educational resources and pointed to AHA Web sites such as the AHA Go Red for Women Web site[49] or the pregnancy and heart disease–Go Red for Women Web site[50] to supplement the education from the obstetrician, gynecologist, or other primary care providers. Lifestyle changes with regular exercise if not already part of the pregnant woman's routine should be encouraged during pregnancy especially for those women who are overweight or obese. The exercise program should be continued postpartum to decrease weight retention and to achieve a healthier adult weight. ACOG supports aerobic exercise and strength conditioning during pregnancy, and the American College of Cardiology/AHA 2013 lifestyle guidelines advocated for 10,000 steps daily for maintenance of heart health.[14,51]

SUMMARY

Multiparity and pregnancy complications confer an increased risk for cardiovascular morbidity and mortality in women. Obesity, excessive weight gain, and weight retention following pregnancy likely adds to the cumulative risk of pregnancy complications of preeclampsia, GDM, prematurity, and low birth for the development of CVD in women and higher risk of mortality compared with men. Pregnancy complications in the past have not been recognized in the AHA guidelines as a risk factor for CVD prevention.[14] To improve the cardiovascular health of women, the obstetrician-gynecologists and women's health care providers, primary care physicians, and cardiologists must ensure that a comprehensive history of pregnancy complications is included for all women at the annual well women's visit. Coordinated care and follow-up for women with pregnancy complications where evidence suggests an increased risk for CVD should focus on education, lifestyle intervention, and early and enhanced cardiac screening with the goal of minimizing cardiovascular morbidity and mortality.

DISCLOSURE

The authors have nothing disclose.

REFERENCES

1. The Global Burden of Disease 2013 Mortality and Causes of Death Collaborators. Global, regional, and national age-sex specific all cause and cause-specific mortality for 240 causes of death, 1990-2013: a systematic analysis for the Global Burden of Disease Study 2013. Lancet 2015;385:117–71.

2. Bots SH, Peters SAE, Woodward M. Sex differences in coronary heart disease and stroke mortality: a global assessment of the effects of ageing between 1980 and 2010. BMJ Glob Health 2017;2:1–8.

3. Yusef S, Hawken S, Ounpuu S, et al, INTERHEART Study Investigators. Effect of potentially modifiable risk factors associated with myocardial infarction in 52 countries (the INTERHEART study); case-control study. Lancet 2004;364:937–52.

4. Heart disease and stroke statistics – 2017 update. A report from the American Heart Association. Circulation 2017;135:e603.

5. Bairey Merz CN, Anderson H, Spague E, et al. Knowledge, attitudes, and beliefs regarding cardiovascular disease in women: The Women's Heart Alliance. J Am Coll Cardiol 2017;70:123–32.

6. Rich-Edwards JW, Fraser A, Lawlor DA, et al. Pregnancy characteristics and women's future cardiovascular health: an underused opportunity to improve women's health? Epidemiol Rev 2014;36(1):57–70.

7. Fraser A, Nelson SM, Macdonald-Wallis C, et al. Associations of pregnancy complications with calculated cardiovascular disease risk and cardiovascular risk factors in middle age. The Avon Longitudinal Study of parents and children. Circulation 2012;125:1367–80.

8. Wenger NK. Recognizing pregnancy-associated cardiovascular risk factors. Am J Cardiol 2014;113:406–9.

9. Wu P, Gulati M, Kwok CS, et al. Preterm delivery and future risk of maternal cardiovascular disease: a systemic review and meta-analysis. J Am Heart Assoc 2018;7:e007809.
10. Carter EB, Stuart JJ, Farland LV, et al. Pregnancy complications as markers for subsequent maternal cardiovascular disease validation of a maternal recall questionnaire. J Womens Health (Larchmt) 2015;24:702–12.
11. Smith GN, Louis JM, Saade GR. Pregnancy and the postpartum period as an opportunity for cardiovascular risk identification and management. Obstet Gynecol 2019;134(4):851–62.
12. Smith GN, Walker MC, Liu A, et al, Hladunewich M for the members of the PE-NET. A history of pre-eclampsia identifies women who have underlying cardiovascular risk factors. Am J Obstet Gynecol 2009;200:58e1-8.
13. Smith GN, Pudwell J, Roddy M. Maternal Health Clinic: a new window of opportunity for early heart disease risk screening and intervention for women with pregnancy complications. J Obstet Gynaecol Can 2013;35(9):831–9.
14. Brown HL, Warner JH, Gianos E, et al. Promoting risk identification and reduction of cardiovascular disease in women through collaboration with obstetricians and gynecologist. Circulation 2018;137:e843–52.
15. Lawlor DA, Emberson JR, Ebrahim S, et al. Is the association between parity and coronary heart disease due to biological effects of pregnancy or adverse lifestyle risk factors associated with child-rearing? Circulation 2003;107:1260–4.
16. Oliver-Williams C, Vladutiu CJ, Loehr LR, et al. The association between parity and subsequent cardiovascular disease in women: the atherosclerosis risk in communities study. J Womens Health (Larchmt) 2019;28(5):721–7.
17. Parikh NI, Lloyd-Jones DM, Ning H, et al. Association of number of live births with left ventricular structure and function. The Multi-Ethnic Study of Atherosclerosis (MESA). Am Heart J 2012;163:470–6.
18. Granger JP, Alexander BT, Llinas MT, et al. Pathophysiology of preeclampsia: linking placental ischemia/hypoxia with microvascular dysfunction. Microcirculation 2002;9(3):147–60.
19. Alnes IV, Janszky I, Forman MR, et al. A population based study of associations between preeclampsia and later cardiovascular risk factors. Am J Obstet Gynecol 2014;211(6):657e.1-7.
20. McDonald SD, Malinowski A, Zhou Q, et al. Cardiovascular sequelae of preeclampsia/eclampsia. A systematic review and meta-analyses. Am Heart J 2008;156(5):918–30.
21. Bellamy L, Casas JP, Hingorani AD, et al. Pre-eclampsia and risk of cardiovascular disease and cancer later in life. Systematic review and meta-analysis. BMJ 2007;335(7627):974.
22. Bassily E, Bell C, Verma S, et al. Significance of obstetrical history with future cardiovascular disease risk. Am J Med 2019;12:567–71.
23. McDonald SD, Ray J, Teo K, et al. Measures of cardiovascular risks and subclinical atherosclerosis in a cohort of women with a remote history of preeclampsia. Atherosclerosis 2013;229(1):234–9.
24. Grandi SM, Filion KB, Yoon S, et al. Cardiovascular disease-related morbidity and mortality in women with a history of pregnancy complications. Circulation 2019; 139(8):1069–79.
25. Drost JD, Arpaci G, Ottervanger JP, et al. Cardiovascular risk factors in women 10 years post early preeclampsia. The preeclampsia risks evaluation in PEMales study (PREVPEM. Eur J Prev Cardiol 2012;19(5):1138–44.

26. Agastisa P, Ness R, Roberts J, et al. Impairment of endothelial function in women with a history of preeclampsia: an indicator of cardiovascular risk. Am J Physiol 2004;286(4):1389–93.
27. Goueslard K, Cottenet J, Mariet AS, et al. Early cardiovascular events in women with a history of gestational diabetes. Cardiovasc Diabetol 2016;15:15.
28. Kjos SL, Peters RK, Xiang A, et al. Predicting future diabetes in Latino women with gestational diabetes. Utility of early postpartum glucose tolerance testing. Diabetes 1995;44(5):586–91.
29. El Ouahabi H, Doubi S, Boujraf S, et al. Gestational diabetes and risk of developing postpartum type 2 diabetes: how to improve follow-up? Int J Prev Med 2019;10:51.
30. Li J, He S, Liu P, et al. Association of gestational diabetes mellitus with subclinical atherosclerosis: a systematic review and meta-analysis. BMC Cardiovasc Disord 2014;14(132):1–9.
31. Sullivan SD, Umans JG, Ratner R. Gestational diabetes: implications for cardiovascular health. Curr Diab Rep 2012;12(1):43–52.
32. Gobl C, Bozhurt L, Yarragudi R, et al. Biomarkers of endothelial dysfunction in relations to impaired carbohydrate metabolism following pregnancy with gestational diabetes. Cardiovasc Diabetol 2014;13:138.
33. Noctor E, Crowe C, Carmody LA, et al. ATLANTIC-DIP: prevalence of metabolic syndrome and insulin resistance in women with previous gestational diabetes by International Association of Diabetes in Pregnancy Study Group criteria. Acta Diabetol 2014;52(1):153–60.
34. Shah BR, Retnakaran R, Booth GL. Increased risk of cardiovascular disease in young women following gestational diabetes mellitus. Diabetes Care 2008; 31(8):1668–9.
35. ACOG Practice Bulletin No. 190. Gestational diabetes mellitus. Obstet Gynecol 2018;131(2):e49–64.
36. Feig DS, Berger H, Donovan L, et al. Canada: a clinical practice guidelines expert committee. Can J Diabetes 2018;42:S255–82.
37. Heida KY, Bots ML, de Groot CJ, et al. Cardiovascular risk management after reproductive and pregnancy-related disorders: a Dutch multidisciplinary evidence-based guideline. Eur J Prev Cardiol 2016;23:1863–79.
38. Bonamy AK, Parikh NI, Cnattinguis S, et al. Birth characteristics and subsequent risks of maternal cardiovascular disease: effects of gestational age and fetal growth. Circulation 2011;124(25):2839–46.
39. Smith GC, Pell JP, Walsh D. Pregnancy complications and maternal risk of ischaemic heart disease: a retrospective cohort study of 129,290 births. Lancet 2001; 357(9273):914–22.
40. Davey Smith G, Whitley E, Gissler M, et al. Birth dimensions of offspring, premature birth, and the mortality of mother. Lancet 2000;356(9247):2066–7.
41. Davey-Smith G, Stern J, Tynelius P, et al. Birth weight of offspring and subsequent cardiovascular mortality of the parents. Epidemiology 2005;16(4):563–9.
42. Catov JM, Wu CS, Olsen J, et al. Early or recurrent preterm birth and maternal cardiovascular disease risk. Ann Epidemiol 2010;20(8):604–9.
43. Rich-Edward JW, Klongsoyr K, Wilcox A, et al. Duration of first pregnancy predicts maternal cardiovascular death, whether delivery was medically indicated or spontaneous (abstract). Am J Epidemiol 2012;175(supl 11):S64.
44. Hastie CE, Smith GC, MacKay DF, et al. Maternal risk of ischaemic heart disease following elective and spontaneous preterm delivery: retrospective cohort study of 750,350 singleton pregnancies. Int J Epidemiol 2011;40(4):914–9.

45. Yu J, Pudwell J, Dayan N, et al. Post-partum breastfeeding and cardiovascular risk assessment in women following pregnancy complications. J Womens Health (Larchmt) 2019. https://doi.org/10.1089/jwh.2019.7894.

46. Schwarz EB, Ray RM, Stuebe AM, et al. Duration of lactation and risk factors for maternal cardiovascular disease. Obstet Gynecol 2009;113(5):974–82.

47. Stuebe AM, Michels KB, Willett WC, et al. Duration of lactation and incidence of myocardial infarction in middle to late adulthood. Am J Obstet Gynecol 2009;200: 138.e1-8.

48. US Preventive Services Task Force Final recommendation statement: high blood pressure in adults: screening. Available at: https://www.uspreventiveservice taskforceorg/page/document/recommendationstatement/high-blood-pressure-in-adults-screening. Accessed February 2020.

49. American Heart Association. Go red for women. Available at: http://www.heart. org/HEARTORG/Causes/Causes_UCM_001128_SubHomePage.jsp. Accessed February 2020.

50. American Heart Association. Go red for women. Pregnancy and heart disease. Available at: https://www.goredforwomen.org/know-your-risk/birth_control_pregnancy_heart_disease/pregnancy-andh-heart-disease. Accessed February 2020.

51. ACOG Committee Opinion No. 650. Physical activity and exercise during pregnancy and the postpartum period. Obstet Gynecol 2015;126:e135–42.

Telehealth in Maternity Care

Haywood L. Brown, MD[a],*, Nathaniel DeNicola, MD, MSHP[b]

KEYWORDS

- Telehealth • Prenatal and postpartum care • Licensing • Credentialing
- Reimbursement

KEY POINTS

- Telehealth and telemedicine can be employed in obstetric practice to facilitate prenatal and postpartum care using various platforms that include videoconferencing and e-medicine.
- Telehealth is governed by the same physician-patient relationships that would be used with a face-to-face encounter, and Internet-based platforms must provide transfer of information that is Health Insurance Portability and Accountability Act compliant.
- The obstetrician-gynecologist and other obstetric providers must address and overcome potential barriers to adopting a telemedicine program, such as connectivity, licensure, legal, credentialing, and reimbursement requirements of states to ensure quality and safe telehealth delivery.

INTRODUCTION

Telehealth involves using digital information and communication technologies, such as computers and mobile devices, to manage health and well-being. Telehealth, also called e-health or mobile health (m-health), includes a variety of health care services. The Centers for Medicare & Medicaid Services define telemedicine as "the use of medical information exchanged from one site to another via electronic communications to improve a patient's health." Telemedicine now is generally thought of as 1 component of telehealth. The World Health Organization defines telehealth as, "The delivery of health care services, where distance is a critical factor, by all health care professionals using information and communication technologies for the exchange of valid information for diagnosis, treatment and prevention of disease and injuries, research and evaluation, and for the continuing education of health care providers, all in the interests of advancing the health of individuals and their communities."[1]

[a] Diversity, Department of Obstetrics and Gynecology, University of South Florida, 13101 Bruce B. Downs Drive, MDC- 3rd Floor, Tampa, FL 33612, USA; [b] Department of Obstetrics and Gynecology, The George Washington University, 2511 I Street Northwest, Washington, DC 20037, USA
* Corresponding author.
E-mail address: haywoodb@usf.edu

Obstet Gynecol Clin N Am 47 (2020) 497–502
https://doi.org/10.1016/j.ogc.2020.05.003
0889-8545/20/© 2020 Elsevier Inc. All rights reserved.
obgyn.theclinics.com

The goal of telehealth is better facilitating care coordination and collaboration, improving quality of care and compliance, fewer hospital admissions and readmissions, fewer face-to-face office visits and cancellations, and improving rural access to care and follow-up in medical and surgical postoperative and postpartum care. Electronic-visits can save patients and doctors time compared with face-to-face office visits. It is of great benefit for those with an established physician-patient relationship and for follow-up care.

One important consideration for telehealth is the use of synchronous versus asynchronous interventions. Synchronous, or real-time, interventions include audiovisual consultations that allow an obstetrician-gynecologist to perform clinical counseling remotely in place of an in-person visit. Real-time audio-visual communication also has been used for clinical scenarios like peer-to-peer consultation, ultrasound imaging review, and directed physical examinations. In other scenarios, the use of asynchronous or store-and-forward telehealth interventions may be more applicable. Some examples of these could include remote monitoring of patient-generated data, such as maternal weight gain and blood glucose, and certain symptom or medical screening questionnaires.[2]

Telehealth is rapidly being adopted into obstetrics and gynecology practice.[2] Telehealth can be helpful especially for obstetric and postpartum care in rural areas and for those who do not have easy access to transportation. Prenatal, intrapartum, and postpartum care in the United States is fragmented between providers and health care facilities that provide obstetric services. This is further compounded by the maldistribution of obstetric providers in the United States.[3] Approximately 6% of the nation's obstetricians and gynecologists practice in rural communities, yet 15%, or approximately 46 million people, live in rural communities. Furthermore, fewer than half of rural women live within a 30-minute drive to the nearest facility providing obstetric services.[4,5]

Access and fragmentation of care for the US obstetric population is further challenged by the fact that 50% of all US hospitals provide care for 3 or fewer deliveries per day. In these situations, identification of risk, team training, and readiness are necessary to address preventable maternal morbidity and mortality.

TELEMEDICINE IN MATERNAL CARE

An example for telemedicine in prenatal care is the program, Text4baby, which utilizes the health belief model by sending cues for positive behavioral and attitude change while providing salient information.

Text4baby is an initiative that seeks to help pregnant women and new mothers increase their knowledge about caring for personal health and giving the infant the best possible start in life.[6] The National Healthy Mothers, Healthy Babies Coalition launched Text4baby, the first free health text messaging service in the United States, in February 2010. Messaging includes information on alcohol and tobacco cessation as well as taking prenatal vitamins and seeking prenatal care. Higher levels of text message exposure changed attitudes and beliefs and predicted lower self-reported alcohol consumption postpartum (odds ratio [OR] 0.212; 95% CI, 0.046–0.973; $P = .046$). The Text4baby program found 40% of enrollees were from underserved zip codes. Additionally, 82% were from households where the yearly income was less than $20,000 per year.[6]

A systematic review of 47 articles that included low-risk and high-risk obstetric, family planning, and general gynecology patient encounters suggests benefit with telehealth interventions, including text messaging and remote monitoring. Text messaging and remote monitoring decrease the number of unscheduled visits.[7]

In 2014, Babyscripts began a program of remote prenatal encounters geared toward transforming how doctors and pregnant women think of and use technology to improve prenatal care. Two landmark studies and partnerships with General Electric, March of Dimes, StartUp Health, and relationships with many of the leading hospitals, health systems, and medical practices around the country have proved to be of benefit in replacing face-to-face prenatal visit encounters for low-risk obstetric patients by monitoring and transmitted blood pressure and weight measurements directly to the prenatal providers, who can incorporate these measurements into the patients' records.[8,9] Remote monitoring for high risk pregnancies with gestational diabetes mellitus also has been included in the platform by providing glucose monitoring and follow-up to providers.

There is a shortage and maldistribution of obstetricians in the United States, particularly in rural communities. Team training is important to provide for readiness to manage preventable morbidity from hemorrhage and for management of hypertension. Through telehealth, regionalized obstetric care relationships and partnerships can be tightened between health centers (clinics), hospitals, and all obstetric care providers: obstetricians, family physicians, advanced practice nurse practitioners, and midwives.

Most recently, through legislation, the state of Texas, in collaboration with the American College of Obstetricians and Gynecologists, established a partnership—Levels of Maternal care verification program.[10] The Maternal Health Compact, published by Mann and colleagues,[11] can be adopted by every facility and community providing obstetric care. The Compact addresses readiness by formalizing relationships between lower-resource hospitals, which may be in rural access communities, to promote the transfer of a pregnant woman who requires a higher level of maternity care. Through telehealth and teleconsultation, the lower-level facility can be connected to the higher-level facility for immediate consultation for an obstetric emergency or anticipated complications, thereby averting the potential for severe morbidity or mortality. For example, a woman diagnosed with placenta previa or invasive placenta disorder would benefit from transfer to a facility capable of dealing with the potential hemorrhage. A woman with a preterm or term preeclampsia with severe features could be transferred when medically stable from a lower-resource facility to a higher-level facility, where hypertension management protocols can be implemented to prevent potential hypertension-related morbidity and cerebral hemorrhage. This communication and support to the clinicians and facilities on the transfer and receiving end of obstetric care define the maternal levels of care that, if universally adopted by all states and facilities, can be an intervention that would lead to reduction in maternal morbidity and mortality.[12]

Emergency obstetric care could be adapted from programs, such as those by Avera e-Care, based in Sioux Falls, South Dakota, for tele-ICU and e-Emergency care throughout the Avera e-Care network of facilities in South Dakota and neighboring states in the network. Emergency obstetrics (tele-Obstetrics) could assist in management of obstetric emergency, such as hemorrhage (pharmacologic and balloon insertion), evaluation of fetal monitoring tracings, and complicated deliveries by nonobstetrician delivery providers (family physicians and midwives) in rural settings, such as those communities in South Dakota where distance and weather can have an impact on immediate transfer of an obstetric patient at risk for morbidity and mortality to a tertiary center.[11]

Postpartum lactation counseling and follow-up can be facilitated through telehealth video encounters, especially for women in rural communities where access to follow-up and resources is challenging. Text communications and Web-based platforms focused on breastfeeding have showed improvement in breastfeeding exclusivity and continuation rates postpartum.[7] These types of encounters can lead to improvement in the disparity in breastfeeding continuation in minority women. Women who are experiencing problems with breastfeeding in the first several weeks postpartum are less likely to continue with exclusive breastfeeding for the recommended weeks and are more likely to discontinue breastfeeding in favor of formula feeding. Connecting with a professional particularly in lactation can provide the encouragement that a woman needs for both maternal and newborn benefit.[7,13]

Telemedicine, specifically telepsychiatry, has been practiced in this country since at least the mid-1960s. In 1964, the Nebraska Psychiatric Institute received a grant from the National Institute of Mental Health to link the Institute with Norfolk State Hospital, more than 100 miles away, by closed-circuit television. Telepsychiatry uses technology to facilitate psychiatric care at a distance and can be used specifically in follow-up for women screened and diagnosed with postpartum depression. Case studies from Australia evaluated the effectiveness of telemedicine as a strategy for providing a broad range of services related to child and adolescent mental health and to improve the accessibility of rural and remote health to specialist child and adolescent mental health consultation and support.[14]

With regard to postpartum depression follow-up, telehealth overcomes the barrier of having to travel to see a specialist and allows for screening in the weeks and months after childbirth to prevent the exacerbation of depressive symptoms. Videoconferencing can be used for check-in visits with a nurse, obstetrician, or other obstetric service provider or with a psychiatric physician or psychotherapist, who can adjust medications as necessary without having the woman travel to an office for a face-to-face encounter.

CHALLENGES IN IMPLEMENTATION OF TELEHEALTH

One of the essential challenges to implementation of telehealth is overcoming network, connectivity, and equipment requirements and expenses required for initiation of a telehealth program. This can be especially of concern in rural clinical and hospital settings where services are most needed to improve access and follow-up. It is important for telehealth providers and facilities to be familiar with the hardware, software, and security requirements to provide quality, safe, and Health Insurance Portability and Accountability Act–compliant care.

Box 1
Telehealth and the physician-patient relationship

Patient-physician relationship
- A patient-physician relationship generally is formed when a physician affirmatively acts in patient care by examining, diagnosing, treating, or agreeing to do so.
- Once a physician consensually enters into relationship with a patient in any of these ways, a legal contract is formed.
- The physician owes a duty to that patient to continue to treat or properly terminate the relationship.

Liability
- Duty of care for patient
- Where is medicine practiced (states)?
- Where is practitioner licensed (states)?
- Is physical contact require?
- Is standard of care applied (patient or doctor)?

Licensing, credentialing, and privileging for telehealth depend on the state(s) and facilities where the services are being provided. Telemedicine parity refers to the equivalent health insurance reimbursement for similar in-person and telehealth services.[15] Thirty-five states have enacted telemedicine parity laws defining reimbursement for fee for services.[16] Rules for patient encounters, documentation, and treatment guidelines should be the same as for face-to-face enounters that govern the physician-patient relationship. Liability insurance policies should cover telemedicine across all states where a physician is providing services (**Box 1**).

SUMMARY

Telehealth and enhanced technology for clinical care and education augment the fragmented model of current prenatal, intrapartum, and postpartum obstetric practice and will enhance quality and safety issues in maternity care. Telehealth is critical to full implementation of Levels of Maternal Care and the Alliance for Innovation on Maternal Health safety bundles to improve quality and safety in care delivery, especially in rural access communities.

Innovation in health care delivery through telemedicine/telehealth is evolving at a rapid speed.

Teleconsultation for inpatient, outpatient, and emergency management is rapidly becoming a modality to improve access and the quality of care in rural and urban settings for all specialties, including obstetrics and gynecology.

Obstacles to implementation of a robust telemedicine program include available technology in many rural settings, cost and reimbursement, and liability concerns.

Postpartum follow-up for all women can be facilitated by embracing technology and telehealth through various platforms and to provide health promotion.

DISCLOSURE

H.L. Brown: Merck for Mother Advisory Board and Up to Date contributor. N. DeNicola has nothing to disclose.

REFERENCES

1. WHO. A health telematics policy in support of WHO's Health-For-All strategy for global health development: report of the WHO group consultation on health telematics, 11–16 December, Geneva, 1997. Geneva (Switzerland): World Health Organization; 1998.
2. Implementing Telehealth in Practice. ACOG Committee opinion number 798 presidential task force on Telehealth. The American College of Obstetricians and Gynecologists 2020;135(2):e73–9.
3. Phelan ST, Wetzel L. Maternal death in rural America. Contemp Ob Gyn 2018;17(8).
4. Marsa L. Labor pains: the ob gyn shortage. AAMC News 2018.
5. Kozhimannil KB, Hung P, Henning-Smith C, et al. Association between loss of hospital-based obstetric services and birth outcomes in rural counties in the US. ACOG guidance: emergency treatment for severe hypertension in pregnancy. JAMA 2018;319(12):1239–47.
6. Whittaker R, Matoff-Stepp S, Meehan J, et al. Text4baby: development and implementation of a national text messaging health information service. Am J Public Health 2012;102(12):2207–13.

7. DeNicola N Grossman D, Marko K, Somalkar S, et al. Telehealth interventions to improve obstetric and gynecologic health outcomes: a systematic review. Obstet Gynecol 2020;135:371–82.
8. Marko KI, Krapf JM, Meltzer AC, et al. Testing the feasibility of remote patient monitoring in prenatal care using a mobile app and connected devices: a prospective observational trial. JMIR Res Protoc 2016;5(4):e200.
9. Marko KI, Ganju N, Krapf JM, et al. A resource and cost analysis on the impact of reduced visits for prenatal care. Obstet Gynecol 2016. https://doi.org/10.1097/01.AOG.0000483884.36730.d5.
10. Texas Levels of Maternal Care Verification Program. Available at: https://www.acog.org/About-ACOG/ACOG-Departments/LOMC/Texas-Levels-of-Maternal-Care-Verification-Program?IsMobileSet=falseBarriers to Breastfeeding in the United States. https://www.ncbi.nlm.nih.gov/books/NBK52688/. Accessed March 29, 2020.
11. Mann S, McKay K, Brown H. The maternal health compact. N Engl J Med 2017; 376:1304–5.
12. Obstetric care consensus No. 2. Levels of maternal care. Obstet Gynecol 2015; 125:502–15.
13. dos Santos LF, Borges RF, de Azambuja Zocche DA. Telehealth and breastfeeding: an integrative review. Telemed J E Health 2019. https://doi.org/10.1089/tmj.2019.0073.
14. Mitchell JM, Robinson PJ, McEvoy M, et al. Two case studies of telehealth technologies used for the delivery of professional development for health, education and welfare professionals in remote mining towns. J Telemed Telecare 2001;7: 174–80.
15. ACOG committee opinion number 798. Implementing Telehealth in Practice. Obstet Gynecol 2020;135:E73–9.
16. Center for Connected Health Policy. State Telehealth Laws and Reimbursement Policies Report. Available at: http://www.cchpca.org/state-laws-and-reimbursement-policies. Accessed March 29, 2020.

Moving?

Make sure your subscription moves with you!

To notify us of your new address, find your **Clinics Account Number** (located on your mailing label above your name), and contact customer service at:

Email: **journalscustomerservice-usa@elsevier.com**

800-654-2452 (subscribers in the U.S. & Canada)
314-447-8871 (subscribers outside of the U.S. & Canada)

Fax number: **314-447-8029**

Elsevier Health Sciences Division
Subscription Customer Service
3251 Riverport Lane
Maryland Heights, MO 63043

*To ensure uninterrupted delivery of your subscription, please notify us at least 4 weeks in advance of move.

Printed and bound by CPI Group (UK) Ltd, Croydon, CR0 4YY

08/05/2025

01864697-0005